Neuroanatomy
for Medical Students

Neuroanatomy
for Medical Students

J. L. Wilkinson O.B.E., M.D., F.R.C.S., D.T.M. & H.
Department of Anatomy, University College, Cardiff

with a Foreword by Sir John Walton

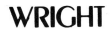

Bristol 1986

Published by
John Wright & Sons Ltd, Techno House, Redcliffe Way, Bristol BS1 6NX.

British Library Cataloguing in Publication Data
Wilkinson, J.L.
    Neuroanatomy for medical students.
    1. Neuroanatomy
    I. Title
611'.8   QM451

ISBN 0 7236 0817 2

Typeset by
BC Typesetting, 51 School Road, Oldland Common, Bristol BS15 6PJ.

Printed in Great Britain by
John Wright & Sons (Printing) Ltd at The Stonebridge Press, Bristol BS4 5NU.

Preface

This textbook is written in response to the needs expressed by preclinical medical students. It is also influenced by many years of medical practice. Preclinical students are advised to retain it for future reference during clinical training; an understanding of the central nervous system's organization is essential to the diagnosis of neurological disorders. Assuming such knowledge, neurology textbooks often have sparse anatomical illustrations; it is hoped that this volume will fill any such gaps. The longest chapter is on the cranial nerves and their disorders, because such palsies are a common clinical problem; for the same reason there is an account of cerebral vascular accidents.

An overall view of the central nervous system is desirable prior to detailed regional study; the introductory section provides a brief account of its gross anatomy based on development. This is followed by a consideration of cell structure, essential to an appreciation of function. The introduction is completed by an account of the peripheral connexions. Thereafter, regional descriptions complement lectures and practical courses in neuroanatomy. Illustrations of dissections and cross-sectional structure assist the latter and each brainstem section combines a photograph and an outline diagram. Coloured illustrations increase printing costs and are therefore limited to Chapters 4–7.

The decision to provide a succinct presentation of information has necessitated a restriction on the amount of current research work which can be described. The chemistry of pathways in the central nervous system is of growing pharmacological interest and my colleague Dr. R. M. Santer has contributed to a concise survey of this subject in the last chapter. Brief accounts are also given of developments in histochemical, immunocytochemical and neuron-tracing techniques; there are clinical references to neuronal plasticity; recent experimental neuron transplantation is mentioned. Phylogenetic considerations, mostly outside the scope of this text, are conducive to an understanding of the motor pathways and of the cerebellum. In this context the prefix arche- (= archae), as in archecerebellum, is used instead of the more usual archi-; together with other nomenclature this conforms with the fourth edition of the *Nomina Anatomica*. Neurophysiological emphasis on Rexed's laminae is tending to displace traditional descriptions of nuclei in the spinal grey matter; aggregations of somata readily visible in human spinal cord sections are described here and related to laminar structure.

I am greatly indebted to Professor Roger Warwick who, although occupied in revising *Gray's Anatomy*, found time to read this manuscript; his editing expertise resulted in a more concise text. The illustrations by our departmental artist Miss Catherine Hemington are a patient and skilful transformation of my inexpert drawings. My thanks are also due to Mr. Peter Hire for his photography and to Miss Julie Broadbent who typed most of the final draft. It has been helpful to discuss this project with colleagues Dr. R. Presley and Dr. R. M. Santer; in addition Dr. J. A. Findlay contributed the photographs in *Fig.* 12.3 and the diagrams in *Figs.* 7.10 and 7.11, and Professor D. B. Moffat the photograph in *Fig.* 7.9. Finally I am grateful to the Publishers and especially to Mr. David Kingham and Mr. R. Lamb for their advice and co-operation.

J. L. W.

Contents

Foreword

Sir John Walton T.D., M.D., D.Sc., M.A., F.R.C.P.
Warden of Green College, Oxford
Formerly Professor of Neurology, University of Newcastle-upon-Tyne
Consultant Neurologist, Newcastle District Hospitals

For many years in medical education descriptive and topographical anatomy has been under attack, with the implication that much of the detail taught to medical students of a generation ago is no longer relevant to modern medical practice. Most clinicians would now accept that many of the minutiae of anatomical interrelationships need not be memorised by the average medical student, even if they are still essential for the specialist surgeon who can acquire this information in his postgraduate training. And I suppose it is only natural that some specialists in clinical disciplines seem to hold the view that cuts in teaching hours in anatomy might most properly be imposed in relation to the structure of anatomical systems other than that with which their clinical specialties are primarily concerned. Not surprisingly, as a neurologist, I am a firm believer in teaching medical students basic neurobiology, which implies that they must achieve a thorough grounding in those principles which are relevant to understanding the structure and function of the nervous system; inevitably this necessitates the acquisition of a core of fundamental knowledge of neuroanatomy. Without such a basis, it is in my view impossible for a doctor to interpret the symptoms and signs of dysfunction of the nervous system in such a way as to construct a differential diagnosis which leads in turn to a planned programme of investigation and treatment in the best interests of his patients.

This book, clearly and succinctly written by Dr Wilkinson, profusely and in my view beautifully illustrated, presents just that basic core of essential knowledge that provides the infrastructure upon which, with accompanying physiological and biochemical information, a stable edifice of neurological pathophysiology can be established. I believe that this background is needed by all doctors intending to work in any form of clinical practice and that, in consequence, many medical students and young doctors, in the course of their undergraduate or postgraduate training, will find Dr Wilkinson's book of very great value.

Chapter 1

Development and topography of the nervous system

DEVELOPMENT

A study of embryology helps to explain the nervous system's organization (*Fig.* 1.1). In the early embryonic disc, ectoderm overlying the newly-formed notochord thickens to form a midline *neural plate*. As somitic mesoderm develops alongside the notochord, the neural plate margins are elevated as folds, creating a *neural groove*. Fusion of these folds extends caudally from the cervical region, creating a *neural tube*, with small openings, the *neuropores*, at its rostral and caudal ends, which close by the end of the fourth intrauterine week. Vertebral bodies develop around the notochord, which persists as a nucleus pulposus in each intervertebral disc. (Incomplete closure of the caudal neuropore and defective development of associated vertebral arches produces *spina bifida*.) At the junctions of the neural plate and general ectoderm are the *neural crest cells*; neural tube formation, together with the process of embryonic segmentation segregates these, initially dorsally and then dorsolaterally, as the primordial dorsal root ganglia. (Other neural crest cells provide neurolemmal sheath cells for spinal nerve fibres or migrate to become sympathetic ganglion cells and chromaffin cells of suprarenal medulla.) The rostral part of the neural tube enlarges into forebrain, midbrain and hindbrain vesicles; the remainder retains its cylindrical shape as the spinal cord, neural proliferation in its walls eventually narrowing the lumen to a minute central canal.

The spinal cord

Transverse sections of the neural tube reveal matrix (ependymal), mantle and marginal zones (*Fig.* 1.1). The inner, *matrix zone* is wide, its numerous cells undergoing mitosis; it produces neuroblasts and spongioblasts, the former developing into neurons, the latter into neuroglial cells (astrocytes and oligodendrocytes). Details of histogenesis are beyond this brief account. The neuroblasts migrate to the adjacent *mantle zone*, the future spinal grey matter; their axons enter the external *marginal zone*, the future white matter. Some central processes from the dorsal root ganglia ascend in the marginal zone, while others synapse with neurons in the mantle zone. When histogenesis is complete, the remaining matrix cells differentiate into ependymal cells lining the central canal.

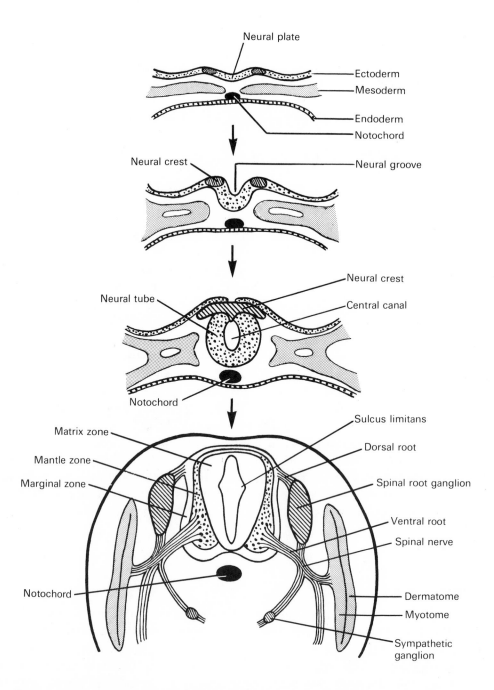

Fig. 1.1 Transverse sections showing progressive differentiation of the neural tube and associated structures.

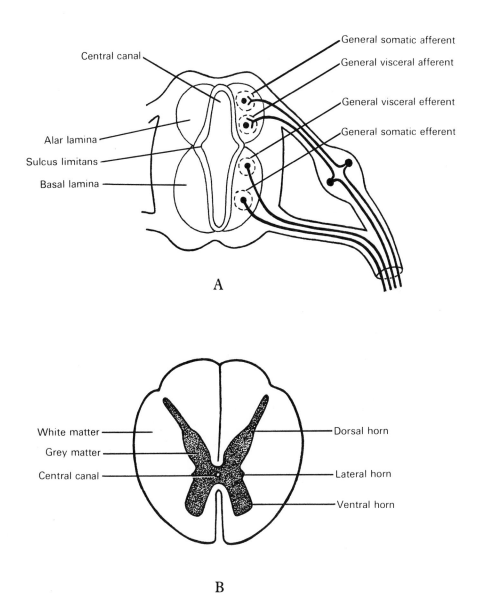

Fig. 1.2 Transverse sections of developing spinal cord showing (A) four cell columns in grey matter, (B) mature (thoracic) spinal cord.

The dorsal and ventral walls of the neural tube remain thin as *roof and floor plates*. On each side the wide mantle zone is demarcated into dorsal and ventral regions by an inner longitudinal *sulcus limitans*; dorsal cells which form the *alar lamina* are functionally afferent, while cells in the *basal lamina* are efferent, their axons leaving the spinal cord as ventral roots which, with peripheral processes of the dorsal root ganglia, form spinal nerves (*Fig.* 1.2).

The alar and basal laminae are subdivided into four longitudinal *cell columns* (seen as 'horns' in cross-section) with specific functions. The two afferent columns of each alar lamina receive axons from the dorsal root ganglia. The *general somatic afferent* column, extending throughout the spinal cord and occupying most of the future dorsal horn, receives impulses from superficial (cutaneous) and deep (proprioceptive) receptors. The *general visceral afferent* column, at the base of the dorsal grey horn in the thoraco-lumbar and sacral regions, receives impulses from the viscera and blood vessels. The *general visceral efferent* column provides preganglionic fibres (synapsing in ganglia) for the viscera, glands and blood vessels; sympathetic outflow is from a thoracolumbar lateral horn, while parasympathetic outflow is via certain cranial nerves and from sacral segments. The *general somatic efferent* column, extending throughout the spinal cord in the ventral horn, innervates skeletal muscle. These four columns are termed 'general' because additional 'special' components exist in the brainstem. Aggregations of nerve cell bodies (*somata*), visible in transverse sections of grey matter, are often referred to as '*nuclei*'; each nucleus has particular functions and its neurons share common pathways.

Initially the spinal cord and vertebral canal are of equal length, but the latter grows more rapidly; at birth its caudal end is level with the third lumbar vertebra and in adults reaches only the disc between the first and second lumbar vertebrae. The more caudal spinal nerve roots are hence elongated and pass obliquely within the canal to emerge via intervertebral foramina; beyond the spinal cord's tip a bundle of lumbar, sacral and coccygeal roots extends caudally to their respective foramina.

Three membranes, derived from mesenchyme, surround the brain and spinal cord; these *meninges* are termed, from within outwards, pia mater, arachnoid mater and dura mater, and will be described later.

The brain

Three brain vesicles, rostral in the neural tube, indicate the early division of the latter into *forebrain* (prosencephalon), *midbrain* (mesencephalon) and *hindbrain* (rhomb-encephalon) (*Fig.* 1.3); their cavities become the ventricular system of the adult. Three flexures appear in this region (*Fig.* 1.4); two are convex dorsally, a *cephalic flexure* (at midbrain level) and a *cervical flexure* (at the junction of hindbrain and spinal cord). A *pontine flexure*, concave dorsally, produced by unequal growth at future pontine level, has a buckling effect, everting the lateral walls and attenuating the roof of the neural tube here (*Fig.* 1.5). The alar laminae (sensory) thus become lateral to the basal laminae (motor) in the floor of a rhomboid-shaped fossa (hence the name rhombencephalon). The part of the hindbrain caudal to the pontine flexure is the *myelencephalon* (future medulla oblongata); the rostral part, from which the pons and cerebellum develop, is

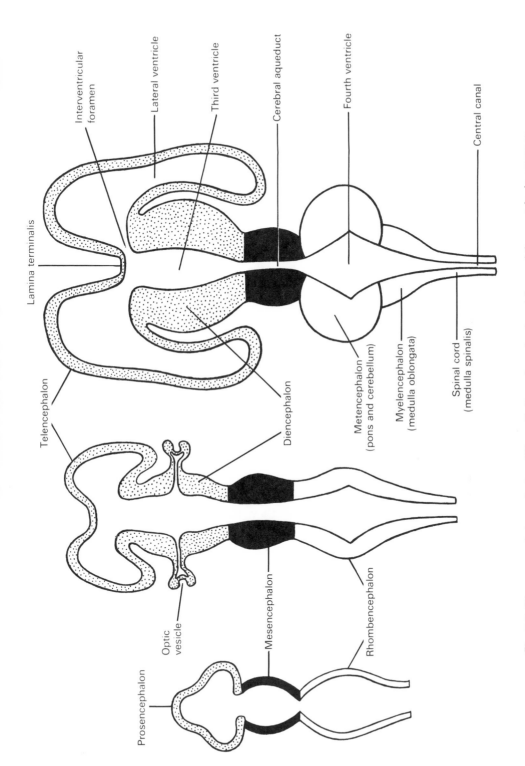

Fig. 1.3 Diagrams of stages in the differentiation of cerebral vesicles and the ventricular system.

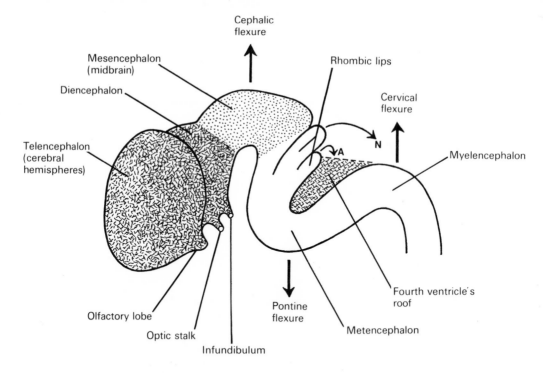

Fig. 1.4 Diagram of the external form of a developing brain and its flexures. Arrows from the rhombic lips indicate the direction of growth of the cerebellum: the neocerebellum (**N**) comes to overhang the fourth ventricle's thin roof, dorsal to the archecerebellum (**A**).

the *metencephalon*; the hindbrain cavity becomes the *fourth ventricle*. In contrast, the narrowed mesencephalic cavity becomes the *cerebral aqueduct*. The forebrain vesicle develops bilateral outgrowths which together constitute the *telencephalon* (= 'end brain'); these overgrow and cover the original forebrain which becomes the diencephalon (= 'between brain'). The twin telencephalic cavities become *lateral ventricles*, while the midline diencephalic cavity becomes the *third ventricle*.

The hindbrain (rhombencephalon)

The caudal myelencephalon has a central canal and becomes the closed part of the medulla. Rostrally this canal widens into the fourth ventricle; its floor, derived from myelencephalon (medulla) and metencephalon (pons), has a longitudinal sulcus limitans on each side, separating the alar and basal laminae. Cranial nerves with nuclear origins in these laminae differ from spinal nerves in the number and type of their components. In addition to four general components, there are special sensory nuclei concerned with taste (gustatory), hearing (cochlear) and equilibration (vestibular), and special motor nuclei innervating muscle of branchial origin. Some cranial nerves have

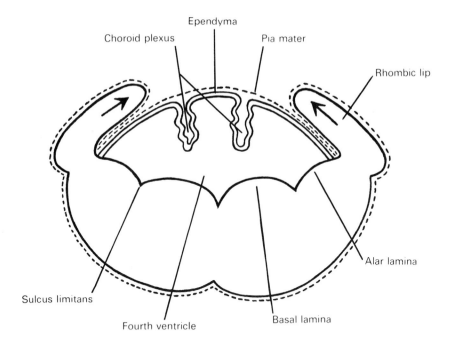

Fig. 1.5 Developing fourth ventricle and cerebellum. Pia mater vascularizes ependyma to form a choroid plexus in the roof. Alar laminae lie lateral to basal laminae. Rhombic lips, derived from alar laminae, grow together to form the cerebellum, dorsal to the ventricular roof.

only one component, either sensory or motor, while others have more, for example the vagus nerve has five. Concerned with input to the developing cerebellum, numerous *pontine nuclei* and the medullary *inferior olivary nucleus* migrate ventrally from the alar laminae. Long ascending and descending fibres ultimately traverse the ventral region.

The attenuated roof of the developing fourth ventricle is a single layer of ependymal cells with a thin covering of pia mater; this is the *tela choroidea*, a vascularized membrane in which a *choroid plexus* of blood vessels forms (*Fig.* 1.5). The fourth ventricle communicates with the subarachnoid space through three apertures, one median and two lateral (*see* p. 74).

The *cerebellum* grows from *rhombic lips*, which are bilateral dorsal extensions of the metencephalic alar plates (*Fig.* 1.5). These meet and fuse over the fourth ventricle's roof and then grow dorsally, folding the tela choroidea and its plexuses inwards towards the ventricular cavity. The neocerebellum, phylogenetically recent and forming much of the cerebellar hemispheres, grows rapidly to overlie the more primitive archecerebellum (*Fig.* 1.4).

The *otocyst*, from which the membranous labyrinth of the internal ear develops, is an invagination of a small area of thickened surface ectoderm (otic placode) on each side of the hindbrain; it becomes isolated from the surface.

The midbrain (mesencephalon)

The mesencephalon retains a generally cylindrical form, its lumen narrowed as the cerebral aqueduct (*Figs*. 1.3, 1.12). The nuclei of two motor cranial nerves (oculomotor and trochlear) develop bilaterally in its basal laminae. Cells of the alar laminae invade the roof plate, forming bilateral longitudinal ridges which later become subdivided by a transverse groove; thus four small elevations, the *corpora quadrigemina*, develop in the tectum (roof) dorsal to the aqueduct. The origins of the red nuclei and substantia nigra (*Fig*. 1.12) are less certain.

The forebrain (prosencephalon)

At an early stage, before closure of the anterior neuropore, paired, hollow, lateral *optic vesicles* diverge forwards from the forebrain. On reaching the surface ectoderm, these invaginate to form retinae, from which nerve fibres grow proximally through the hollow optic stalks to form optic nerves.

The *diencephalon* develops from the original forebrain vesicle. The bilateral *thalami* form in dorsal regions of the third ventricle's walls, the *hypothalamus* in their lower regions and floor. A downgrowth from the floor, the *neurohypophysis*, joins an upgrowth from the stomodeum which becomes the *adenohypophysis*; together these constitute the *hypophysis cerebri* (pituitary gland). The roof plate consists only of ependyma and pia mater anteriorly; as in the fourth ventricle, this forms a *tela choroidea* with *choroid plexuses*. The *epithalamus*, consisting of the pineal gland and habenular nuclei, develops posteriorly in the roof plate. The closed rostral end of the neural tube persists as a thin *lamina terminalis*.

The *telencephalon* comprises paired cerebral vesicles on each side of the lamina terminalis, each communicating with the third ventricle through an interventricular foramen. The telencephalon, developing as two cerebral hemispheres, enlarges upwards, forwards and backwards, its caudal growth enclosing the diencephalon on each side (*Fig*. 1.6). The lowest part of its two medial walls remains merely as ependyma and pia mater; these become the bilateral *choroid fissures*, extending posteriorly from each interventricular foramen, through which the tela choroidea and choroid plexus of the third ventricle invaginate into each lateral ventricle (*Fig*. 1.7). Immediately above each choroid fissure, a thickening of the medial wall forms the *hippocampus*, phylogenetically ancient (archecortex); the two hippocampi are connected by the *fornix*. Subsequent massive development of the cerebral hemispheres (neocortex) displaces the hippocampi posteroinferiorly, the fornix being drawn out as an efferent tract on its medial aspect. The choroid fissure also becomes curved, interposed between fornix and diencephalon.

Commissural fibres interconnect the growing hemispheres and initially the only median structure which can be bridged is the lamina terminalis (*Fig*. 1.7). The *anterior commissure* develops in, and remains connected to, the lamina terminalis, passing from the olfactory bulbs and temporal lobes of one hemisphere to those of the other. The *corpus callosum*, the major interhemispheric commissure, also starts in the upper lamina terminalis but, together with the hemispheres, it expands posteriorly, lying above the

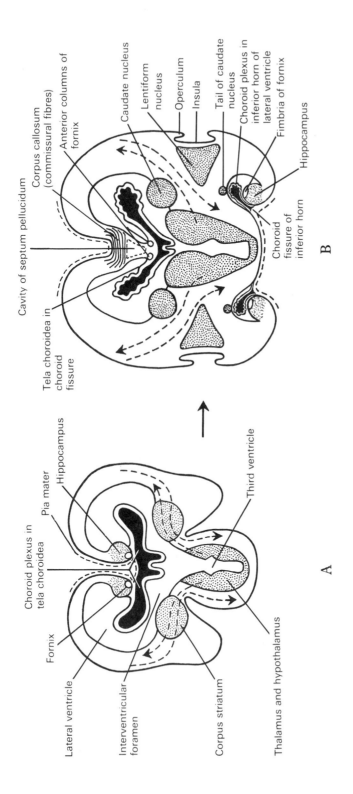

Fig. 1.6 Coronal sections through forebrain to show development of the internal capsule. Arrows indicate the path of developing projection fibres. In (A) there is invagination of choroid plexuses into the lateral and third ventricles. In (B) fusion has occurred between the lateral surfaces of the diencephalon and the ventromedial aspects of the enlarging telencephalon; corpus callosum has separated tela choroidea from dorsal surface; ependyma and residual pia mater form a septum pellucidum with small central cavity; the hippocampus has been displaced inferiorly; the choroid fissure extends from interventricular foramen to inferior horn of lateral ventricle.

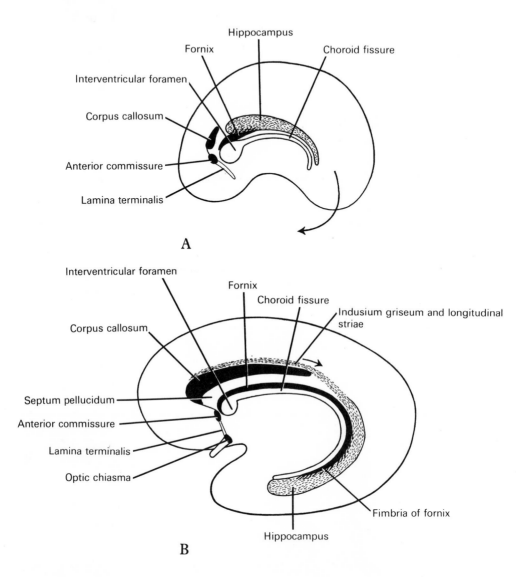

Fig. 1.7 Medial aspects of foetal cerebral hemispheres to show development of commissures and the choroid fissure. In (A) the corpus callosum is rudimentary and the hippocampus overlies the interventricular foramen. In (B) the hippocampus is being displaced into the developing temporal lobe; its fornix bounds the choroid fissure peripherally.

fornix and connected to it by a thin midline *septum pellucidum*. Thus the corpus callosum invades the areas formerly occupied by the hippocampi; vestigial hippocampal remnants remain on its superior surface as a very thin mantle of grey matter, the *indusium griseum*, embedded in which are white *longitudinal striae*. The pia mater of the diencephalic roof is continuous anteriorly with that under the corpus callosum; as the latter extends posteriorly, the two pial layers fuse in the tela choroidea, whose plexuses project into the third and lateral ventricles. Between the caudal edge of the developing corpus callosum and the posterior diencephalic roof (epithalamus), the two pial layers separate at the *transverse cerebral fissure*, via which choroidal arteries enter and internal cerebral veins leave (*Fig.* 1.9).

The *corpus striatum* develops in the telencephalon's floor bilaterally, its margins adjacent to the thalami (*Fig.* 1.6) (primitively these areas of grey matter are sensorimotor 'control centres'). Meanwhile, a major pathway must develop for descending fibres from the cortex and ascending fibres from the thalamus to the cortex; the only route is through this region. Hence these fibres, which form the *internal capsule* on each side, divide the corpus striatum into a dorsomedial *caudate nucleus* which bulges into the lateral ventricle, and a ventrolateral *lentiform nucleus* which is deep to the cortex (here known as the *insula*).

The *cerebral hemispheres* grow rapidly forwards (frontal region), posteriorly (occipital region), then anteroinferiorly (forming the temporal lobe). This curved pattern of expansion from the interventricular foramina round the diencephalon explains the C-shaped formation of related structures such as the lateral ventricles, choroid fissures and fornix (*Fig.* 1.7). Each caudate nucleus has a cauda or tail which curves round into the temporal lobe. Initially the cortical surface is smooth. At the end of the third intrauterine month a lateral depression appears over each lentiform nucleus; rapid growth in adjoining areas causes a *lateral cerebral fissure* to develop here, the submerged cortex forming the insula. With continued development the cortical surface becomes furrowed by *sulci*, the intervening convolutions forming *gyri*. Neuroblasts develop in the deep (matrix) zone and migrate superficially into the cortex, the intervening zone becoming white matter.

GENERAL TOPOGRAPHY IN THE ADULT

The *central nervous system* comprises the brain and spinal cord; the *peripheral nervous system* comprises the cranial and spinal nerves and their ramifications.

Peripheral nervous system

There are 12 paired cranial and 31 paired spinal nerves. The constituent nerve fibres innervate somatic or visceral structures and convey afferent (sensory) or efferent (motor) impulses. *Somatic efferent fibres* pass directly from their cells of origin in the central nervous system to skeletal muscle. *Autonomic (visceral) efferent fibres* from the central nervous system are pre-ganglionic, that is they synapse in peripheral ganglia with neurons which innervate non-striated muscle and glands. *Somatic and autonomic afferent fibres* pass from peripheral receptors to their cells of origin in the spinal dorsal root ganglia, or in the equivalent ganglia of certain cranial nerves; as the first stages of a relay to the brain they are *primary sensory neurons*.

The autonomic nervous system has *sympathetic* and *parasympathetic* divisions. Sympathetic outflow is from the spinal *thoracolumbar* region (T1–L2). Parasympathetic outflow is *craniosacral* in origin, occurring from two widely separated sources, via the oculomotor, facial, glossopharyngeal, and vagus cranial nerves and the second, third and fourth sacral spinal nerves. Sympathetic and parasympathetic systems generally have opposing actions. Sympathetic activity accompanies expenditure of energy, as in an emergency situation ('fright, fight, flight') producing such symptoms as pupillary dilatation, cardio-acceleration, cutaneous vasoconstriction, increased blood pressure, reduced peristalsis and contraction of sphincters. Parasympathetic activity conserves and restores energy ('repose and repair'), slowing the heart rate and increasing peristalsis and glandular activity.

Central nervous system

The brain and spinal cord may be described (in a rather simplified way) as consisting of grey matter (nerve cell bodies and mostly non-myelinated fibres) and white matter (chiefly myelinated fibres) with neuroglial cells occurring throughout. Topographically the central nervous system may be divided into forebrain (cerebrum and diencephalon), midbrain, hindbrain (pons, medulla oblongata and cerebellum) and spinal cord (medulla spinalis). The midbrain, pons and medulla oblongata collectively form the *brainstem*.

The forebrain

The *cerebrum* consists of paired hemispheres which occupy the anterior and middle cranial fossae. Each has an external grey *cortex* and a white centrum; in the latter there are deep grey masses, the *basal ganglia*. The two hemispheres are partly separated by a deep median longitudinal fissure, crossed by a massive commissure, the *corpus callosum*, whose fibres interconnect corresponding cortical areas. The cerebral cortex is convoluted by *gyri* and furrowed by *sulci*; the *insular cortex* is submerged in the *lateral fissure* (of Sylvius); the *central sulcus* extends from the superomedial border of the hemisphere, slightly posterior to its mid-point, down and forwards towards the lateral fissure. Sulci partially divide the hemispheres into lobes named after the cranial bones adjacent to them (*Fig.* 1.8). The *frontal lobe* is anterior to the central sulcus and above the lateral fissure; the *parietal lobe* is posterior to the central sulcus and above the lateral fissure; the *occipital lobe* is behind a line from the parieto-occipital sulcus to the pre-occipital notch; the *temporal lobe* is below the lateral fissure and in front of the pre-occipital notch. The so-called *limbic lobe* is a composite bordering zone (limbus) between the telencephalon and diencephalon, extending through the septal area (anterior to the lamina terminalis) and the cingulate gyrus (above the corpus callosum) to the parahippocampal gyrus (on the inferior surface of the temporal lobe, adjacent to the brainstem and continuous with the hippocampus).

The *diencephalon*, lying between the cerebral hemispheres and the brainstem, consists of thalami, hypothalamus and epithalamus. Each *thalamus*, an ovate nuclear mass lateral to the third ventricle, is a major relay and integration centre for ascending fibres, receiving axons of secondary sensory neurons in the spinal cord and brainstem; thalamic tertiary sensory neurons project to the cerebral cortex. The thalami also integrate motor functions, relaying impulses from the cerebellum and corpus striatum to the motor cortex. Connexions with the limbic system influence behaviour, mood and memory. The *hypothalamus* (= 'below thalamus') regulates visceral activity through the autonomic nervous system and hormonal activity through the hypophysis cerebri. The *epithalamus*, posterosuperiorly, includes the pineal gland and habenular nuclei. Reduction of pineal secretion precipitates puberty; the habenular nuclei have olfactory and limbic connexions. The *subthalamus* lies between the diencephalon and the mesencephalon.

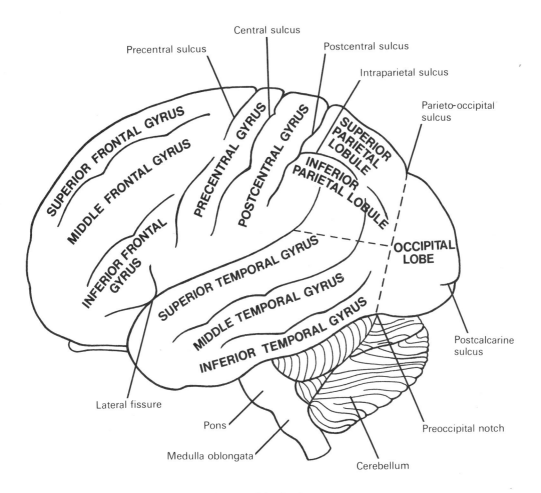

Fig. 1.8 Lateral aspect of the left side of the brain.

The basal ganglia include the corpora striata and the mesencephalic substantia nigra and red nuclei; relaying through the thalamus to the cortex, they influence the quality of motor performance and are sometimes termed 'extrapyramidal nuclei'. The red nuclei also have caudal connexions. During development of connexions between the cortex and the brainstem, bundles of fibres, converging as the *internal capsules*, partially divide each corpus striatum into a medial caudate and a lateral lentiform nucleus (*Figs.* 9.2, 9.4). Between the internal capsule and the cortex, nerve fibres diverge as the *corona radiata*.

Within each cerebral hemisphere a *lateral ventricle* has a central body, anterior horn (in the frontal lobe), posterior horn (in the occipital lobe) and inferior horn (in the temporal lobe) (*Fig.* 1.10). It connects via an *interventricular foramen* with the third ventricle, which continues via the cerebral aqueduct to the fourth ventricle. Cerebrospinal fluid, formed by ventricular *choroid plexuses*, passes through apertures in the fourth ventricle into the subarachnoid space around the brain and spinal cord. The two lateral ventricles are separated by the *septum pellucidum* between the corpus callosum and the fornix, seen in a sagittal section (*Fig.* 1.9). Each interventricular foramen is bounded behind by the thalamus and in front by the fornix and anterior commissure.

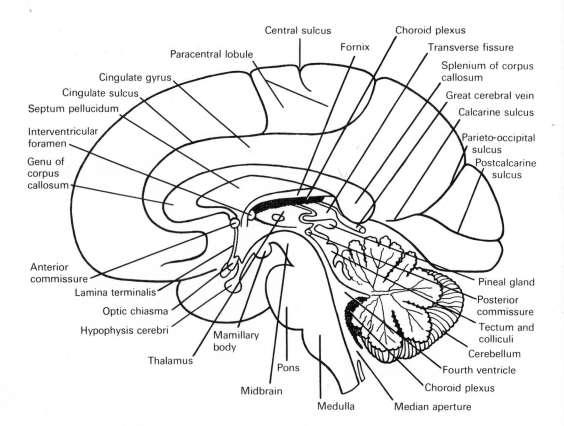

Fig. 1.9 Median sagittal section of the brain.

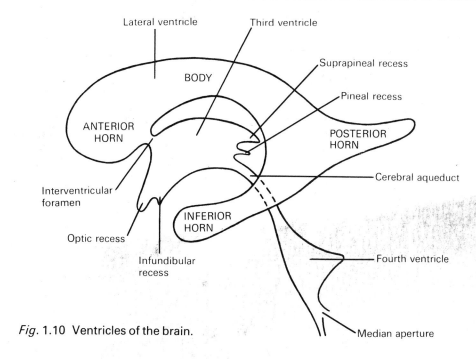

Fig. 1.10 Ventricles of the brain.

The brain and spinal cord are surrounded by three *meninges*, the pia mater, arachnoid mater and dura mater. The *pia mater* is adherent to the brain and spinal cord, conveying small arteries into their substance. The subarachnoid space (between pia mater and arachnoid mater) contains cerebrospinal fluid and the major arteries; the latter may rupture and produce 'subarachnoid haemorrhage'. The *dura mater* adheres to the internal cranial surface, and is infolded vertically between the cerebral hemispheres as a sickle-shaped *falx cerebri* (*Fig.* 13.1). The *tentorium cerebelli* is a horizontal dural partition over the posterior cranial fossa and between the cerebrum and the cerebellum, its free edge at midbrain level. The dura mater encloses *venous sinuses* which receive blood from the brain.

The midbrain

The *mesencephalon* (*Figs.* 1.9, 1.12) is traversed by the *cerebral aqueduct*; the *tectum*, dorsal to this, has four surface elevations, the *corpora quadrigemina* (comprising two superior and two inferior colliculi). Ventral to the aqueduct are the *cerebral peduncles*, consisting of a central *tegmentum* separated ventrally from two *crura cerebri* by pigmented grey matter, the *substantia nigra*. Each crus, in continuity ipsilaterally with the internal capsule, contains fibres descending to the spinal cord (corticospinal fibres), pontine nuclei (corticopontine fibres) and brainstem (corticobulbar fibres). Between the crura is the *interpeduncular fossa*. In the tegmentum are two large, oval, pinkish, nuclear masses, the *red nuclei*. Each *superior cerebellar peduncle* enters the lower midbrain; its fibres decussate (cross over), some passing into a red nucleus, most ascending to the thalamus. The oculomotor and trochlear cranial nerves have midbrain origins.

The hindbrain

The *rhombencephalon* consists of pons, medulla oblongata and cerebellum. The pons is continuous above with the midbrain and below with the medulla oblongata, which blends into the spinal cord (medulla spinalis) just below the foramen magnum (*Fig.* 1.11). The hindbrain cavity is the fourth ventricle.

The *pons* is a broad bridge, its transverse fibres forming the *middle cerebellar peduncles*; an anterior median sulcus adjoins the basilar artery. In transverse section (*Fig.* 1.12) it is seen to consist of a large ventral and a smaller dorsal region. Ventrally there are bundles of descending fibres; from numerous *pontine nuclei* transverse fibres form the opposite middle cerebellar peduncle. In the dorsal part, or *tegmentum*, is a diffuse *reticular formation* of small cells and fibres (which extends throughout the brainstem) and nuclei of the trigeminal, abducent, facial and vestibulocochlear cranial nerves.

The *medulla oblongata* (*Figs.* 1.9, 1.11, 1.12) is somewhat conical, its caudal closed part and central canal continuous with the spinal cord; rostrally the canal opens into the

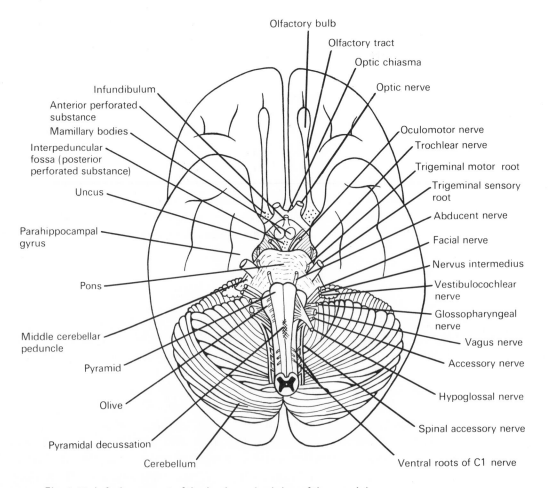

Fig. 1.11 Inferior aspect of the brain and origins of the cranial nerves.

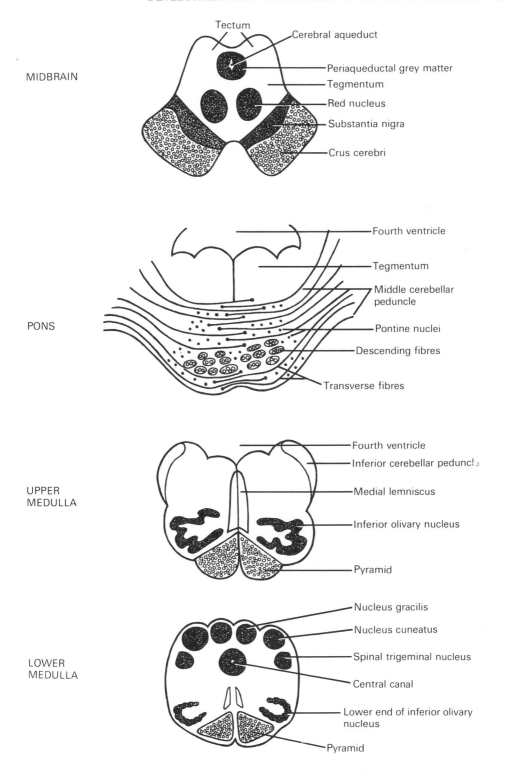

Fig. 1.12 Transverse sections of the brainstem.

fourth ventricle. Bilateral ventral elevations, the *pyramids*, contain corticospinal (pyramidal) fibres, most of which cross in a *pyramidal decussation* to descend contralaterally in the spinal cord. Lateral to each pyramid an oval surface swelling, the olive, contains the *inferior olivary nucleus*, where various cerebellar afferents converge. Dorsal to each olive is an *inferior cerebellar peduncle*. On the dorsal medullary aspect are bilateral *cuneate and gracile tubercles* produced by similarly named nuclei which receive dorsal column spinal fibres. The medulla contains nuclei of the glossopharyngeal, vagus, cranial accessory and hypoglossal cranial nerves. The trigeminal sensory nuclear complex extends throughout the brainstem and into the first two spinal cord segments.

The *cerebellum*, dorsal to the pons and medulla, has two lateral *hemispheres* and a midline *vermis*. It is connected respectively to the midbrain, pons and medulla by superior, middle and inferior *peduncles*. The *cortex* has narrow transverse *folia* (leaf-like in sections), separated by deep fissures. The white medullary centre contains *intracerebellar nuclei*, the largest being the *dentate nucleus*. The cerebellum is close to the fourth ventricle's roof, formed by *superior and inferior medullary vela*, the latter invaginated by a choroid plexus and perforated posteriorly by a median aperture. The ventricular floor (rhomboid fossa) has a recess on each side, leading to two lateral apertures.

The spinal cord

The spinal cord is continuous rostrally with the medulla oblongata and ends caudally as a tapered *conus medullaris*, level with the first lumbar intervertebral disc (between L1 and L2) in adults. The dura mater, arachnoid mater and the *subarachnoid space* (containing cerebrospinal fluid) extend to vertebral level S2. External to the dura mater an *epidural space* contains fat, blood vessels and lymphatics.

Cervical and lumbar enlargements of the cord are associated with limb innervation. The region of origin of a pair of spinal nerves marks a *cord segment*. The paired spinal nerves are: 8 cervical, 12 thoracic, 5 lumbar, 5 sacral and 1 coccygeal, each attached by a dorsal (sensory) and a ventral (motor) root. The spinal nerves pierce the dura mater, traverse the epidural space and leave the vertebral canal through intervertebral foramina. The lumbar, sacral and coccygeal nerve roots extend beyond the spinal cord as the *cauda equina*, which resembles a horse's tail.

The spinal cord has central grey and peripheral white matter. In transverse sections grey matter has an irregular H-shape (*Fig.* 1.2) with two *ventral horns*, two *dorsal horns* and a *grey commissure* containing a minute *central canal*. In the thoracic and upper lumbar regions there are also *lateral horns*. These horns are grey columns in the intact cord. White matter is divided bilaterally into *ventral, lateral and dorsal white columns* (*funiculi*) by the lines of attachment of spinal nerve roots.

Chapter 2

Neurons and neuroglia

THE NEURON

Neurons are cells specialized for the reception and transmission of information. Each has a cell body or *soma* and processes or *neurites*. Receptor neurites, known as *dendrites*, are usually numerous, while each soma has one efferent process, the *axon*. The cytoplasm or *perikaryon* of the soma contains perinuclear basophilic material in the form of granular *Nissl bodies* which are, however, absent close to the axonal origin in the *axon hillock*. Axons have an external plasma membrane, the *axolemma*, enclosing their cytoplasm, known as *axoplasm*; they may have *collateral branches* and end by *synapses* either with other neurons or with effectors at neuromuscular or neuroglandular junctions.

Neuronal somata vary in size from 5 μm to 120 μm. According to their dendritic patterns they are classified as unipolar, bipolar and multipolar (*Fig. 2.1*). *Unipolar neurons* (e.g. in dorsal root spinal ganglia) have a spherical soma and a single process which bifurcates to pass centrally and peripherally; sometimes termed *pseudo-unipolar*, each develops from a bipolar cell whose processes fuse near the soma. *Bipolar neurons* have an elongated soma with a process at each pole; associated with some special senses, they exist in the retina, the olfactory mucosa and the cochlear and vestibular ganglia. *Multipolar neurons*, afferent or efferent, are irregular in somal shape with many dendrites and are the most numerous central neurons; they are classified as Golgi Type I or II. *Golgi Type I neurons* have a large soma and a long axon, for example pyramidal cells of the cerebral cortex, Purkinje cells of the cerebellar cortex and spinal ventral horn cells. *Golgi Type II neurons* are small, often stellate, with an axon terminating locally, for example interneurons.

Neurocytological investigation

For light microscopy, neural tissue may be stained in various ways. *Nucleic acid dyes*, including cresyl violet and toluidine blue, stain nuclei and Nissl bodies, demonstrating somata but not axons. *Silver stains* (e.g. *Cajal* and *Golgi* methods) depend on the affinity of neural tissue for silver; nerve cells and their processes stain darkly while myelin is unstained. *Myelin stains*: (a) in the *Weigert* method, potassium dichromate makes myelin sheaths stainable by haematoxylin and they become dark blue; (b) the *Marchi* technique

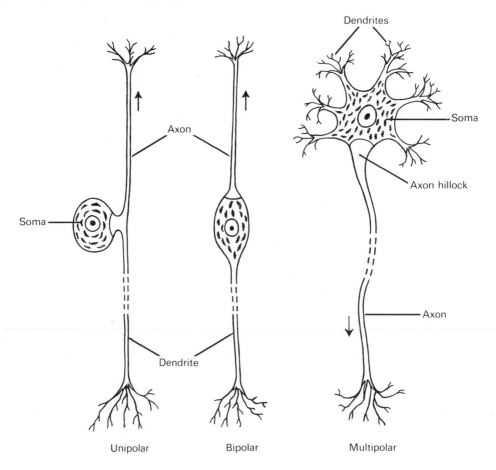

Fig. 2.1 Three basic types of neuron. Arrows indicate the usual direction of impulse transmission.

demonstrates degenerating fibres, potassium dichromate rendering normal myelin yellow-brown, osmic acid staining fatty acids of degenerating myelin black.

In recent years, *histochemical and immunocytochemical techniques* have made possible the identification of individual neurotransmitters and associated enzymes in neurons. For example, using formaldehyde-induced fluorescence, noradrenaline (norepinephrine) appears pale green and serotonin (5–HT) yellow when exposed to ultraviolet light. Neurons have been classified using this method.

Axon-tracing in the past depended on degeneration techniques. If central connexions are destroyed, the axons degenerate; following axonal damage the soma undergoes *chromatolysis*, it swells, the nucleus becomes eccentric in position, and the Nissl bodies disintegrate and are dispersed as fine granules (*Fig. 2.2*). This is the *acute reaction*; after 14 days the cells may show signs of recovery or may die if the axon is damaged near its origin. By removing individual ocular muscles, thereby severing their nerves, Warwick (1953) was able to define their central representation by mapping the resultant chromatolytic neurons. Recent methods have utilized orthograde or retrograde axonal

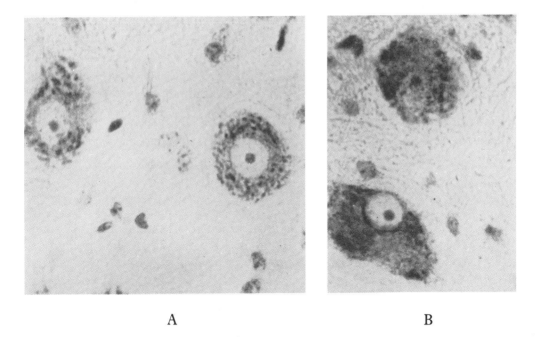

A   B

Fig. 2.2 Chromatolysis in the oculomotor nuclear complex. (A) Normal somatic motor neurons with uniformly distributed large discrete chromatin granules and central nuclei. (B) Following resection of one extra-ocular muscle, somata of affected neurons show disintegration and dispersal of granules and eccentricity of nuclei. (Cresyl violet stain, × 690.) (From an illustration by Warwick R. (1953) *J. Comp. Neurol.* **98**, 499, reproduced by kind permission of author and publisher.)

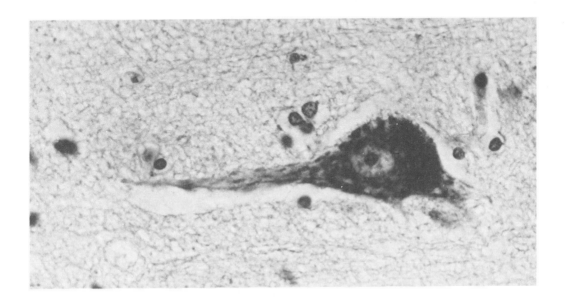

Fig. 2.3 Giant pyramidal (Betz) cell of cerebral motor cortex. (Cresyl violet stain, × 630.)

transport (Cowan & Cuénod, 1975). Uptake by somata of injected radioactive-labelled amino acids and their subsequent distal (orthograde) axonal transport may be traced by autoradiography. An injection of the enzyme horseradish peroxidase (HRP) is taken up by axon terminals or damaged axons and transferred to somata, where it can be identified histochemically.

Electron microscopy has greatly increased detailed knowledge of cell membranes, organelles, synapses and myelin sheath structure. In combination with other techniques, synaptic relationships between identified neurons are now being elucidated at the ultrastructural level.

Cytology (*Fig.* 2.4)

The cell membrane is a complex bilaminar structure of phospholipid and protein molecules with an external layer of glycoprotein. It is semipermeable; in the resting state, potassium ions diffuse out from the cytoplasm, creating a negative resting potential of about -70 mV. Excitation selectively alters membrane permeability, a sudden influx of sodium ions following; this reversal of cell polarity results in an *action potential* or nerve impulse in the axon. Graded potentials of multiple sub-threshold stimuli summate to an 'all or none' response. The impulse, lasting about 5 ms, is followed by a return to the resting potential as potassium ions flow out and then by a *refractory period* during which the cell is unresponsive to stimuli.

The *nucleus* has a double membrane with pores. Its *chromatin* consists of large molecules of deoxyribonucleic acid (DNA), which regulates ribonucleic acid (RNA) synthesis. RNA probably leaves via the *nuclear pores* and controls cell protein synthesis in the ribosomes. There is usually a single *nucleolus*. In females there is a *nucleolar satellite* (Barr body) of sex chromatin. Some binucleate somata appear in sympathetic ganglia.

Cytoplasmic organelles

Nissl bodies (chromatin granules), intensely basophilic and stained by cresyl violet and similar dyes, occupy the perikaryon and dendrites but not the axon hillock (*Figs.* 2.1, 2.3). They are more prominent in motor than in sensory neurons, amounts varying with cell activity. With electron microscopy they are seen to consist of *granular (rough) endoplasmic reticulum*, consisting of stacked cisternae with attached and free ribosomes containing RNA and concerned in production of proteins necessary for cell maintenance, neurotransmitter synthesis and storage.

Golgi complexes, which are clusters of flattened cisternae near the nucleus and similar in appearance to agranular (smooth) endoplasmic reticulum, enclose protein and carbohydrates in membrane-bound vesicles for axonal transport. They also produce *lysosomes*, which are membrane-bound enzymes, able to destroy intracellular bacteria or other foreign material and to dispose of effete intracellular organelles.

Mitochondria, numerous throughout soma, dendrites and axon, are spherical, ovoid or filamentous, with a double membrane folded internally into cristae. Regarded as the 'powerhouse' of cells, they store energy in adenosine triphosphate (ATP). They are particularly evident at sites of metabolic activity, for example near synapses and motor and sensory endings.

Electron microscopy reveals *neurotubules*, 20–30 nm in diameter and composed of the protein tubulin, running through the perikaryon into the neurites; these are concerned with the transport of large molecules along the neurites in either direction. In addition there are *neurofilaments*, about 10 nm thick. Neurotubules and neurofilaments aggregate in silver-stained preparations to form the 'neurofibrils' which are visible in light microscopy.

Centrosomes (centrioles), usually a feature of dividing cells, have been observed in mature neurons incapable of division; they may be associated with the formation or maintenance of neurotubules.

In addition to organelles, *cytoplasmic inclusions* may appear in neurons. *Melanin*, most evident in the substantia nigra, increases in amount up to puberty, then remains constant; it is chemically related to the neurotransmitter dopamine which is utilized by neurons located there. The pontine nucleus caeruleus (caeruleus = dark blue) contains

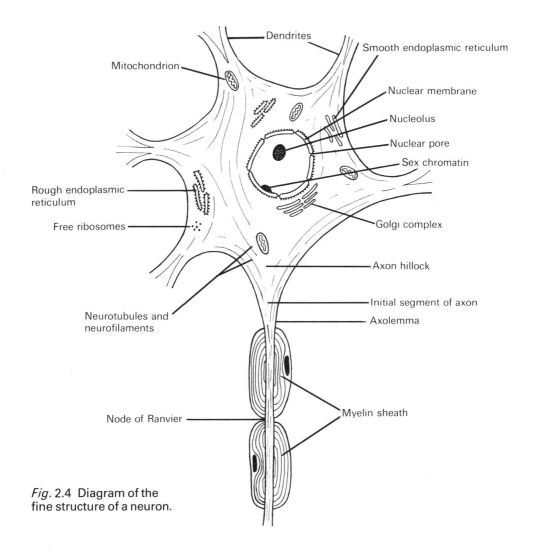

Fig. 2.4 Diagram of the fine structure of a neuron.

melanin and copper. With increasing age, most neurons develop yellowish-brown *lipofuscin* ('age pigment') granules.

Dendrites and axon

Dendrites are slender extensions from the soma which greatly increase the soma's receptive field and contain the same organelles. They commonly have numerous branches whose configurations characterize neuron types (*Fig.* 12.1), for example the Purkinje cells of the cerebellar cortex have a dendritic field arranged in one plane, transverse to the folium (*Fig.* 7.6). Frequently their surface area is extended by synaptic *dendritic spines*.

A single *axon*, generally the longest neurite, usually arises from an *axon hillock* (where action potentials develop); this narrows into an *initial segment*, beyond which the diameter remains uniform. Axons thicker than 1 μm generally have a *myelin sheath* which commences after the initial segment and is interrupted at intervals by the nodes of Ranvier (*see* p. 31). In the central nervous system myelin sheaths are formed by neuroglia (oligodendrocytes), in peripheral nerves by neurolemmal cells of Schwann. At the nodes, the bare axolemma is exposed to ionic exchange, while the myelinated segments (internodes) are insulated; this arrangement is the structural basis for '*saltatory conduction*', by which action potentials 'jump' from node to node. The speed of conduction is proportional to the thickness of the axon and its sheath. Slender axons are non-myelinated. *Collateral branches* arise at nodes, a recurrent collateral recurving towards the parent soma and synapsing with nearby neurons. The *axon terminals* have presynaptic expansions (*boutons terminaux*), or a row of many such swellings (*boutons de passage*). The *axoplasm* contains neurotubules, neurofilaments, agranular (smooth) endoplasmic reticulum and mitochondria; RNA and ribosomes, concerned with protein synthesis, are usually absent from the axoplasm.

Axoplasmic transport

Products synthesized in the soma travel along the axon in the *orthograde* direction in two modes: bulk flow of axoplasm, including mitochondria, at about 1–3 mm/day is relatively *slow transport*. *Rapid transport* of membrane-bound vesicles, including neurotransmitters, has a velocity of about 400 mm/day (2,800 mm/day in the hypothalamo-hypophysial tract); transport probably occurs on the external surfaces of the neurotubules. *Retrograde transport* provides a feedback whereby information on peripheral activity is relayed to the soma. It is used experimentally in axon-tracing (e.g. by horseradish peroxidase) and has a clinical implication in centripetal invasion by neurotoxic and infective agents (e.g. tetanus toxin and rabies). Such mechanisms are still under investigation.

Synapses (Fig. 2.5)

Each neuron is an anatomical unit; this was proposed by Cajal at the end of the ninteenth century, but was finally proven only by electron microscopy. Unidirectional communication occurs at foci of specialized contact, the *synapses*, each occurring between the axon of one neuron and the cell surface of another. Myelinated axons lose their sheaths near their terminals. Each axon may have thousands of boutons; similarly each neuron may be contacted by a few terminals or by thousands, some excitatory, some inhibitory. This general pattern provides for discrete, convergent or divergent transmission of information. The commonest synapse is between an axon and the soma or dendrites of another neuron (*axosomatic, axodendritic*); less common are synapses for inhibitory impulses from one axon to the initial segment or terminal of another (*axoaxonic*). Neurons also synapse with *effectors* at neuromuscular and neuroglandular junctions.

In the central nervous system most synapses are of the type called *chemical synapses*, in which the *presynaptic* and *postsynaptic membranes* are separated by a *synaptic cleft* about 20 nm wide. The presynaptic membrane may have local thickenings, the postsynaptic a dense *subsynaptic web*; these, together with other variable factors, such as width of cleft or type and shape of vesicles, are used in classifying synapses. A presynaptic terminal has *synaptic vesicles* which contain neurotransmitter substance. Arrival of nerve impulses at a terminal creates an influx of calcium ions, which causes release of neurotransmitter by exocytosis into the synaptic cleft, where it unites with *receptors* of the postsynaptic membrane. In excitatory synapses depolarization follows, in inhibitory synapses hyperpolarization of the postsynaptic membrane occurs. The neurotransmitter acetylcholine is inactivated in the cleft by acetylcholinesterase. Catecholamines such as noradrenaline are located in dense-cored vesicles, and the duration of their

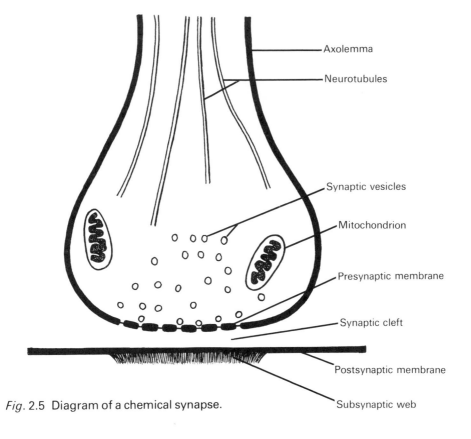

Axolemma

Neurotubules

Synaptic vesicles

Mitochondrion

Presynaptic membrane

Synaptic cleft

Postsynaptic membrane

Subsynaptic web

Fig. 2.5 Diagram of a chemical synapse.

postsynaptic effect is limited by their re-uptake to the presynaptic terminal as well as by enzymatic means. Other transmitters include serotonin (5–HT), dopamine, gamma aminobutyric acid (GABA), glycine, glutamic and aspartic acids, and possibly some peptides, such as substance P.

Electrical synapses, common in invertebrates, may occur in mammals. A narrow *gap junction*, 2 nm wide, contains small channels between apposed membranes, which effect rapid direct transmission of impulses by ionic flow. Gap junctions are like those in cardiac and nonstriated muscle.

NEUROGLIA

Neurons are surrounded by more numerous, non-excitable glial cells, comprising about half the volume of the central nervous system. Unlike neurons, they are able to divide. There are several varieties.

Astrocytes (*Fig.* 2.6), the most numerous, are stellate, with many processes which contact non-synaptic neuronal surfaces, and have 'perivascular feet' which cover 85% of the surface of capillaries within the central nervous system. They form an external glial membrane under the pia mater and an internal membrane under the ventricular ependyma. Their cytoplasm contains bundles of filaments. There are two main sub-types: *fibrous astrocytes*, in white matter, have long slender processes and many filaments; *protoplasmic astrocytes*, in grey matter, have shorter, flattened, branched processes with few filaments. They support neurons, structurally and functionally. When damaged, they hypertrophy and proliferate to form a 'glial scar'. A so-called 'blood/brain barrier' is primarily due to tight junctions between capillary endothelial cells, but astrocytes probably also contribute a selective nutritive path between blood vessels and neurons. They also occur in the retina (cells of Muller). Astrocytes are the commonest source of primary malignant tumours in the central nervous system.

Oligodendrocytes differ in having a smaller, denser nucleus, fewer processes (oligos = few) and no cytoplasmic filaments. *Interfascicular oligodendrocytes*, arranged along myelinated axons, have processes forming myelin internodes on several adjoining axons; in peripheral nerves there is one neurolemmal Schwann cell to each internode. *Perineuronal satellite cells* surround somata. Both types of oligodendrocyte may have nutritive functions, possibly related to high oxygen need.

Microglia, small, irregular cells with a few branched processes, are normally inactive but, like connective tissue macrophages, can become phagocytic.

Ependyma lines the cerebral ventricles and the central canal of the spinal cord (*Figs.* 2.7, 13.8); a single layer of cuboidal cells, its surface may have microvilli and cilia. Subjacent to it is the internal limiting membrane of astrocytes. Embryonic ependyma has more than one cell layer (*Fig.* 2.7), with processes extending through the width of the neural tube to the external limiting membrane. *Choroidal epithelium*, modified for active and selective secretion of cerebrospinal fluid (CSF), is convoluted, its surface further extended by microvilli. Tight intercellular junctions form a 'blood/CSF barrier'; the cell cytoplasm has numerous mitochondria, Golgi complexes and endo-plasmic reticulum. Specialized ependymal cells, *tanacytes*, in the third ventricle's floor, extend from the hypothalamic median eminence to the hypophysial portal system.

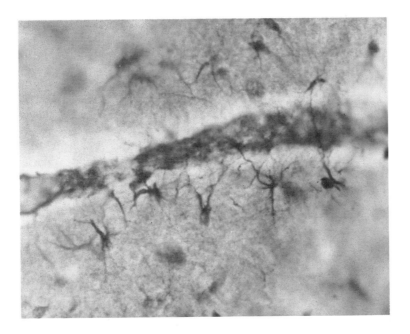

Fig. 2.6 Perivascular astrocytes in the cerebral cortex.
(Bielschowsky silver preparation, × 1000.)

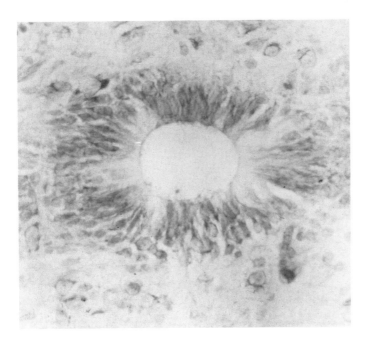

Fig. 2.7 Ependymal cells lining central canal of spinal cord in a chick embryo. The canal's dark outline represents tight junctions between adjacent cells. At this stage of development the ependymal surface is ciliated. Pale-staining neuroblasts are visible in the surrounding mantle zone. (Toluidine blue stain, ×460.)

Chapter 3

Peripheral nervous system

Impulses enter and leave the central nervous system via the cranial and spinal nerves. Cranial nerves may be motor, sensory or mixed; they may be purely somatic or mostly visceral in distribution. The spinal nerves, formed by dorsal and ventral roots, are segmentally arranged; the intercostal nerves, in their cutaneous and muscular supply to the *dermatomes* and *myotomes*, retain the primitive pattern. The dermatomes are prolonged into the limbs but still retain a general numerical sequence except at axial lines (*Fig.* 3.1). The division and redistribution of the embryonic myotomes into individual muscles and their segmental innervation is much more complicated, as the following generalizations indicate. Most muscles are supplied from two segments (although the intrinsic muscles of the hand are unisegmental). Muscles sharing a common primary action are supplied by the same segments, opposing muscles by segments in sequence with the former. Thus in elbow movements, spinal cord segments C5 and 6 supply flexors and C7 and 8 supply extensors. The emergence of motor skills and the evolution of functionally specialized muscles in mammalian limbs required an interchange of fibres from segmental spinal nerves in the brachial, lumbar and sacral *plexuses*, from which plurisegmental nerves enter the limbs. Moreover there is a correlation between the supplies to joints, muscle and skin: *Hilton's Law* states that those 'nerves whose branches supply the groups of muscles moving a joint furnish also a distribution of nerves to the skin over the insertions of the same muscles and the interior of the joint'. In addition to primary segmental interchange in large plexuses, there are secondary *intraneural plexuses* of fibres in plurisegmental nerves within which appropriate branches are formed. This has implications in nerve injuries, since even the loss of a few millimetres renders accurate reapposition impossible.

STRUCTURE OF PERIPHERAL NERVES

Peripheral nerves comprise fasciculi of nerve fibres, myelinated and non-myelinated, enclosed in three sheaths of connective tissue. The nerve trunks are surrounded by *epineurium*, fasciculi by *perineurium* and individual nerve fibres by *endoneurium* (*Fig.* 3.2). Capillaries and lymphatics ramify in this connective tissue. Major arterial occlusion in the limbs may cause severe pain due to ischaemic neuritis.

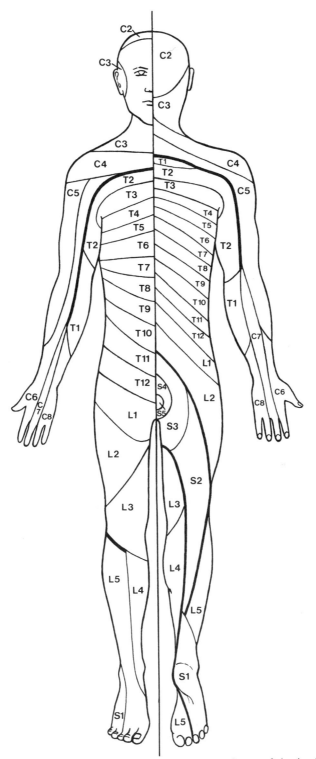

Fig. 3.1 Dermatomes on the anterior and posterior surfaces of the body. Axial lines, where there is numerical discontinuity, are drawn thickly.

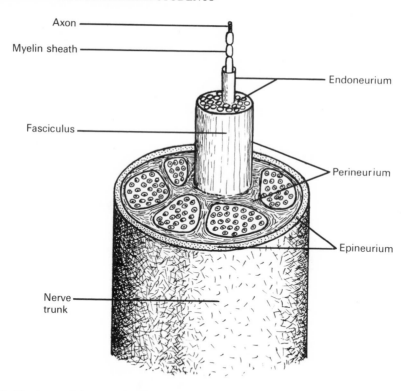

Fig. 3.2 Diagram of the structure of a peripheral nerve.

Classification of nerve fibres

According to axonal diameter (including the myelin sheath if present) and to the speed of conduction, nerve fibres may be divided into three main groups, A, B and C; group A, large and myelinated, are further classified into somatic sensory (I, II, III) and motor (α, β, γ) sub-groups. In the following list, maximum diameters and conduction rates are in brackets.

Afferent A fibres:

Group I: from annulospiral endings of muscle spindles (Ia) and tendon organs (Ib) (20 μm, 120 m/s).

Group II: from 'flower-spray' endings in muscle spindles, touch and pressure receptors (15 μm, 90 m/s).

Group III: from pain and temperature receptors (7 μm, 30 m/s).

Efferent A fibres:

α *fibres:*   supply skeletal (extrafusal) muscle (17 μm, 120 m/s).

β *motor fibres:* few in number, supply extrafusal muscle and muscle spindles.

γ *fibres:*   supply intrafusal muscle (of muscle spindles) (8 μm, 30 m/s).

B fibres: myelinated, preganglionic autonomic (3 μm, 15 m/s).

C fibres: non-myelinated, postganglionic autonomic, also visceral and somatic
                    afferents for pain and temperature sensations (1.5 μm, 2 m/s).

Myelinated and non-myelinated nerve fibres *(Fig. 3.3)*

During development, axons growing peripherally from the ventral column neurons and
the dorsal root ganglia unite to form segmental spinal nerves; they are accompanied at
regular intervals by peri-axonal *Schwann cells*.

Small fibres, usually 1 μm or less in diameter, remain *non-myelinated*, and several
invaginate the plasma membrane of a single Schwann cell. Action potentials travel
continuously along the axolemma, not by the more rapid saltatory conduction, in the
absence of nodes of Ranvier.

Myelinated fibres have a regularly segmented *myelin sheath* interrupted by *nodes of
Ranvier*, each myelinated *internode* being up to 1 mm long. Myelin sheaths begin to
develop before birth but are not complete until a year or more later; a neurolemmal
Schwann cell spirals round an axon, its plasma membrane forming concentric lamellae,
which by electron microscopy appear to consist of a major dense line, where two inner
protein layers of plasma membrane are in apposition, and a less dense double thickness
of lipid, in which a thin intraperiod line represents fused outer membrane surfaces (*Fig.
3.3C*). The cytoplasm and nucleus of the Schwann cell are peripheral in the *neurolemma*;
only a very thin collar of cytoplasm remains next to the axon. The most external and
internal infoldings of the plasma membrane form a *mesaxon*. *Myelin incisures* (of
Schmidt-Lanterman) are regular spiral zones in the sheath where cytoplasm penetrates
centrally between the myelin layers towards the axon. Nodes of Ranvier separate
consecutive sections of the myelin sheath, whose lamellae here form terminal loops
(*Fig. 3.3*). In peripheral nerves the neurolemma extends onto the node, while in the
central nervous system the axolemma is more exposed. Action potentials jump from
node to node by the process called *saltatory conduction*, giving greater velocity
(particularly in large axons with long internodes) than in non-myelinated fibres.

Ganglia

Sensory ganglia on spinal dorsal roots and some cranial nerves have a connective tissue
capsule continuous with the epineurium and perineurium. The somata of primary
sensory neurons, 20–100 μm in size, are mostly peripheral, their processes lying
centrally in the ganglion. They are *unipolar*, a single process bifurcating to pass to
peripheral receptors and to the central nervous system. The peripheral process,
conducting towards the soma, is functionally a dendrite but has the structural and
physiological characteristics of an axon. Impulses pass directly from the peripheral to
the central process, bypassing the soma. *Satellite cells* surround each soma, separating it
from capillaries; they are nutritive and are structurally like neurolemmal cells.

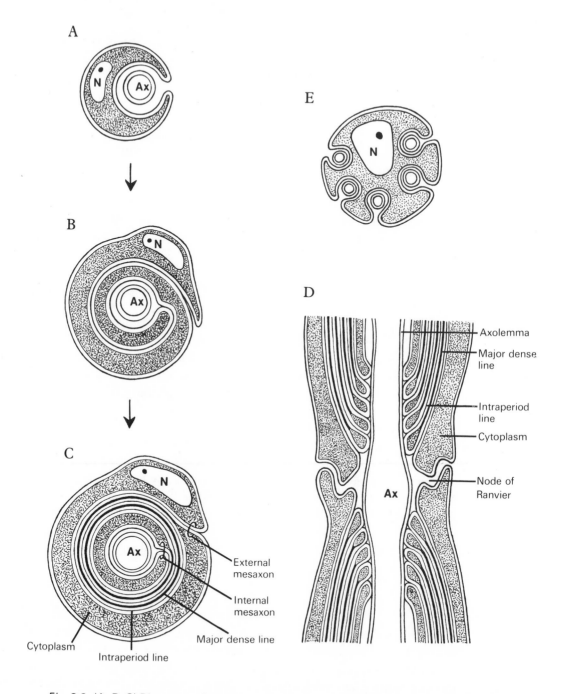

Fig. 3.3 (A, B, C) Diagrams of stages in development of a myelinated sheath. Schwann cell cytoplasm is stippled and its nucleus (**N**) shown; **AX**, axon. (D) Longitudinal section of a myelinated nerve showing fine structure of node of Ranvier. (E) Several non-myelinated axons are related to one Schwann cell.

Autonomic ganglia are situated in the paravertebral sympathetic chains, prevertebral thoracic and abdominal plexuses (e.g. cardiac, pulmonary, coeliac, mesenteric) and in visceral walls. Structurally and functionally they differ from sensory ganglia, being visceromotor and containing synapses. The postsynaptic (principal) cells are multipolar, uniform in size, smaller than many cells in the sensory ganglia, sometimes binucleate and their axons are non-myelinated. There are also interneurons near synapses. Somata and nerve fibres are intermingled. Some myelinated preganglionic fibres traverse the paravertebral ganglia to synapse more peripherally; the afferents also are 'fibres of passage', their somata lying in dorsal root ganglia (*see also* p. 43).

DEGENERATION AND REGENERATION AFTER INJURY

Damage affects nerves both proximally and distally. The soma, the trophic centre of the neuron, undergoes *chromatolysis* (p. 20). From the site of injury *retrograde degeneration* of each axon and its myelin sheath spreads proximally only to the first node and this is quickly followed by regeneration. Distally, *Wallerian degeneration* affects the whole nerve fibre; its axon disintegrates, its myelin sheath breaks into lipid droplets. Schwann cells then proliferate to fill the endoneurial tube, emerging from its cut end.

The soma begins to recover after about three weeks, swelling subsides, Nissl bodies reappear, and the nucleus returns to a central position. Much earlier, within twenty-four hours after injury, axons in the proximal stump start to regenerate. Successful restoration is greatly influenced by the nature of the injury; if the nerve is crushed, the endoneurial tubes may remain intact, and axons may then reach their original territories; when a nerve is severed this is much less likely.

Following section, totally accurate reapposition of cut ends is most unlikely; destruction of only a few millimetres of nerve renders this impossible, because constituent fibres change orientation in a plexiform fashion throughout its length; proliferating axons are unable to cross a major gap and become entangled in a 'stump neuroma'. Local events such as haemorrhage, infection and fibroblastic proliferation may inhibit successful repair. In mixed nerves, somatic, autonomic, motor and sensory fibres may travel to inappropriate endings. Proximal axons develop multiple sprouts and are guided along Schwann cells into the distal, severed parts of endoneurial tubes. Several sprouts from different axons may enter one tube (*Fig.* 3.4), but only one will establish effective contact with the peripheral receptor or effector organ, thicken and remyelinate. In a mixed nerve regeneration of non-myelinated fibres may be poor and vasomotor control imperfect.

Axons may grow as much as 5 mm/day but functional recovery is generally estimated at 1.5 mm/day; crossing the site of injury entails delay, as does establishing effective peripheral contact, thickening and remyelinating. Functional recovery is often incomplete; apart from the factors mentioned, recovery is affected by the length of fibre to be restored and by the ability of atrophied muscle, sense organs and stiff joints to recover. If, for example, the sciatic nerve is severed, the recovered power in the calf muscles may be only 50%; 'foot drop', due to weakness of extensors, persists in most cases and sensory recovery in the foot is usually limited to pain and deep sensation.

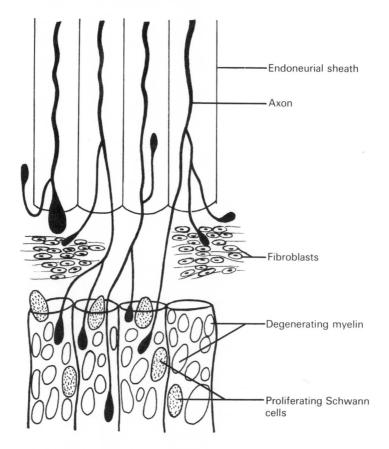

Fig. 3.4 Diagram showing axonal regeneration following nerve severance.

If a nerve is only partly divided, some recovery is due to development of *collateral sprouts* from intact fibres, a marked feature in autonomic nerves. If intentional section (e.g. sympathectomy, vagotomy) is incomplete, the long-term results may hence be disappointing.

RECEPTORS AND EFFECTORS

Receptors

Receptors are transducers, converting mechanical and other stimuli into electrical impulses. They are classified as superficial *exteroceptors* responding to external stimuli, deeper *proprioceptors* stimulated by movement, pressure and change of body position and *interoceptors* from viscera and blood vessels. They may be either *encapsulated* by connective tissue or *unencapsulated* (free or expanded).

Cutaneous receptors (Figs. 3.5, 3.6)

Free nerve endings. Finely myelinated group A (III) and non-myelinated C fibres form subcutaneous and intradermal plexuses, whose rami terminate as naked axons between cells. They are the only type of nerve ending present in the central cornea or in dental pulp. Often regarded as 'pain fibres', they are the most widely distributed receptors and also serve more general functions, including thermal sensation. *Peritrichial* expanded endings occur in the outer root sheath of hair follicles and are stimulated by light touch causing movement of hairs. One nerve fibre supplies many follicles; each follicle is supplied by several myelinated fibres, which lose their sheaths and form a peritrichial plexus. *Tactile discs* (of Merkel) are expanded nerve endings in the germinative epidermal layer of hairless skin. They contact *Merkel cells*, which are specialized epithelial cells with a lobulated nucleus and cytoplasmic secretory granules near the nerve terminal.

Encapsulated nerve endings. Lamellated (Pacinian) corpuscles (*Fig.* 3.6) are the largest and most numerous encapsulated receptors. Ovoid, up to 4 mm long, they have an

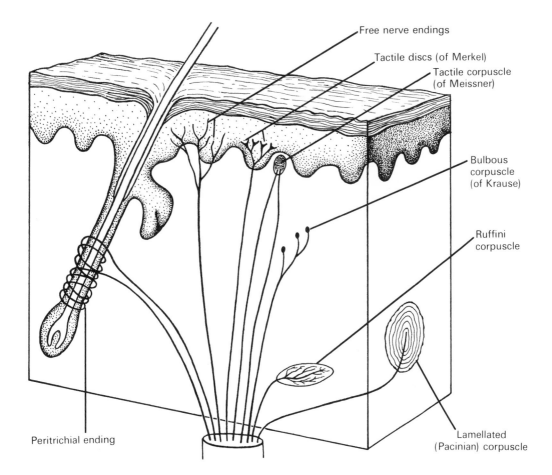

Fig. 3.5 Sensory nerve endings and receptors in the skin.

outer multilaminated capsule of flat cells, and have a myelinated nerve fibre which loses its sheath to enter the central core. They respond to pressure and vibration. *Tactile (Meissner's) corpuscles* are ovoid, about 100 µm long, sited in the dermal papillae and most numerous in the fingertips. They contain transversely arranged epithelioid cells; each corpuscle is supplied by up to four myelinated nerve fibres. Sensitive to tactile stimuli, they probably serve close spatial ('two point') discrimination. *End bulbs* of various types consist of multiple branched nerve terminals, encapsulated: the *bulbous corpuscles* (of Krause), found mainly at mucocutaneous junctions, are spherical and up to 50 µm in diameter; slightly different *genital corpuscles* (of Golgi-Mazzoni) occur in the genital skin.

The primary sensations (modalities) of touch, pain, cold and warmth are represented in the skin by a pattern of spots, each specific to one of these; for example a 'cold spot'. This is not explicable simply by an equivalent local distribution of specific receptors. An individual receptor *and its nerve fibre(s)* respond to only one modality. Thus various free nerve endings may respond to differing stimuli, for example pain or temperature. There

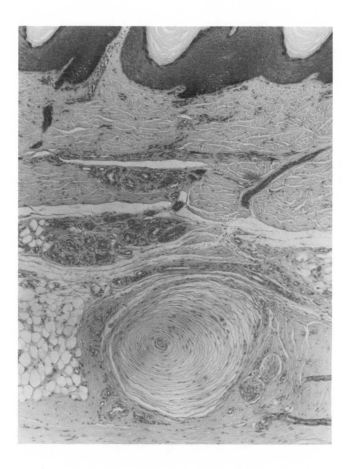

Fig. 3.6 Lamellated (Pacinian) corpuscle in the skin. (Haematoxylin and eosin stain, × 8.)

are two types of pain; 'fast pain' is a sharp pricking sensation involving A (III) fibres, while 'slow pain' is longer lasting and burning in quality and is mediated by C fibres. Central processing of painful stimuli is discussed later (p. 57). Touch and pressure sensations are served by more heavily myelinated A fibres. Complex stimuli may involve several types of receptor; perception presumably requires abstraction, correlation and analysis of the resultant impulses, but the nature of this is largely speculative.

Muscle receptors

The receptors of *neuromuscular spindles* (*Fig.* 3.7) respond to stretch and have essential motor functions. Up to 8 mm long, the spindles consist of specialized *intrafusal* muscle fibres, motor and sensory endings, in a fluid-filled fusiform capsule, orientated parallel to the surrounding (extrafusal) muscle. They are attached at each pole to intramuscular connective tissue; thus when a muscle lengthens, the spindles are stretched. The intrafusal muscle fibres are slender, with cross-striations only at each end; centrally

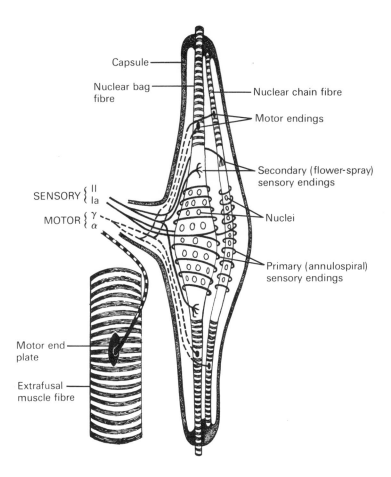

Fig. 3.7 A neuromuscular spindle. Note the innervation of nuclear bag and nuclear chain intrafusal fibres. Motor nerves are shown as interrupted lines.

many nuclei are arranged in sarcoplasm, either in a chain formation (*nuclear chain fibres*) or in an expanded equatorial zone (*nuclear bag fibres*). Nuclear bag fibres are thicker and longer than chain fibres, projecting beyond the capsule at each end and attached to extrafusal connective tissue.

There are two types of sensory ending, termed annulospiral and flower-spray. *Annulospiral (primary) endings* surround the equator of intrafusal fibres and come from thickly myelinated (Type Ia) nerves; they respond rapidly, transmitting information on velocity of change as well as length (dynamic response). *Flower-spray (secondary) endings* are located some distance from the equator, mostly on nuclear chain fibres; they are terminal varicosities of more thinly myelinated (Type II) nerves and respond more slowly, measuring only length (static response).

Extrafusal muscle is innervated by ventral column α motor neurons. Smaller, γ motor neurons terminate at the striated poles of intrafusal fibres. Neuromuscular spindle receptors act either in a passive role (stretch reflex), or actively by initiating the contraction of extrafusal muscle (γ reflex loop) (*Fig.* 4.7). The stretching of extrafusal muscle stimulates the spindle receptors and, via a spinal reflex arc, impulses to α neurons cause contraction of extrafusal muscle, this in turn reducing intrafusal tension. This is a mechanism which is essential for the control of muscle tone and the maintenance of posture. In the γ reflex loop upper motor neurons at cranial level activate spinal γ neurons, intrafusal muscle contracts, spindle receptors respond and, through spinal reflex connexions to α motor neurons, extrafusal muscle contracts, in turn reducing intrafusal tension. This servo-type system enables skeletal muscle to contract in relation to the predetermined spindle length.

Tendon and ligament receptors

Neurotendinous fusiform receptors (of Golgi), up to 500 μm long, are most numerous near musculotendinous junctions. A fusiform capsule contains slender and cellular intrafusal tendon fibres, innervated by group Ib nerves with bulbous terminals. Excitation requires a tension greater than that to which muscle spindles respond. Through spinal interneurons tendon receptors are inhibitory to α motor neurons, thus preventing excessive tension, and balancing excitatory input from neuromuscular receptors. Tendons and ligaments also have free (pain) nerve endings.

Joint receptors

Free nerve endings, profuse in synovial membrane and articular capsules, react to painful stimuli. *Ruffini corpuscles* and *lamellated (Pacinian) corpuscles* in capsules respond to movement and pressure. *Neurotendinous spindle receptors* prevent excessive stretch of the capsular ligaments. Awareness of joint position is largely dependent on neuromuscular spindle receptors.

Receptors in muscles, tendons, joints and ligaments participate in spinal reflexes; they also provide information to the cerebellum (subconscious proprioception) and cerebrum (conscious proprioception or *kinaesthesia*).

Effectors

Somatic effectors are the terminals of ventral column myelinated axons which pass without interruption from the spinal cord to striated muscle. Visceral effectors are supplied by non-myelinated axons from cells in the autonomic ganglia.

Somatic effectors

A single motor neuron and the muscle fibres innervated by it constitute a *motor unit*, which may include hundreds of muscle fibres in large muscles such as gluteus maximus. Where movements are very precise, as in extra-ocular muscles and intrinsic hand muscles, the motor units are small. Having branched a few or many times, an axon ends centrally on each muscle fibre at a *neuromuscular junction* or motor end plate (*Fig.* 3.8). The myelin sheath is lost from the final branches, which are covered by neurolemmal Schwann cells and endoneurium; the former are superficial but are not interposed at the end plate, the latter blends with the endomysium. The expanded, naked, axonal terminal is apposed to the *sole plate* of a muscle fibre; here the sarcolemma forms a 'synaptic gutter', many junctional folds increasing the surface area of this *subneural apparatus*. The axolemma and sarcolemma are separated by a synaptic cleft of 20–50 nm. The terminal axoplasm has mitochondria and synaptic vesicles containing

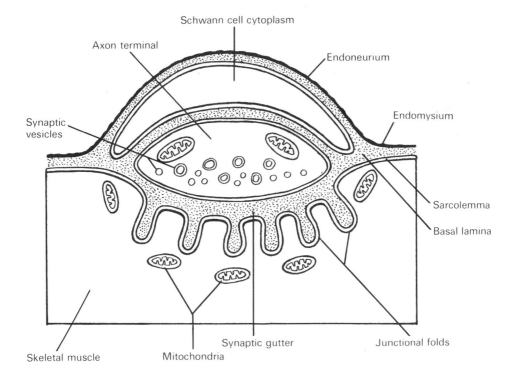

Fig. 3.8 Diagram of a skeletal neuromuscular junction (motor end plate). Between Schwann cell, axon and muscle there is a basal lamina (stippled).

acetylcholine; the subneural apparatus has acetylcholine receptors on the apices of the junctional folds, its sarcoplasm containing many nuclei, mitochondria and acetyl-cholinesterase, which inactivates acetylcholine. Nerve impulses cause exocytosis of the presynaptic vesicles into the synaptic cleft and acetylcholine then binds to postsynaptic receptors and depolarizes the sarcolemma, creating an action potential. Muscle contraction ensues, limited in duration by the action of acetylcholinesterase.

Visceral effectors

Postganglionic fibres are non-myelinated. Where precision and speed are required, as in the iris, innervation is discrete; in enteric muscle, where peristalsis is slow and diffuse, the fibres form plexuses with much branching, each neuron supplying many muscle fibres. There are no specialized endings as in striated muscle; a naked varicose axon terminal, its neurolemmal cytoplasm retracted, occupies a shallow groove in the plasma membrane of cardiac or visceral muscle, and these endings are more widely separated than in skeletal muscle. The terminals are similar in glands. By electron microscopy axoplasmic membrane-bound vesicles of cholinergic terminals (containing acetyl-choline) are clear, while adrenergic terminals (containing noradrenaline) are dense.

AUTONOMIC NERVOUS SYSTEM

The general functions of sympathetic and parasympathetic nerves have been briefly described in Chapter 1; their distribution is shown in *Figs*. 3.9, 3.10. Details of the parasympathetic components in cranial nerves are provided in Chapter 6.

Visceral afferents

Physiological impulses travel mainly in parasympathetic fibres, while nociceptor impulses travel via sympathetic pathways.

Baroreceptors in the carotid sinus and aortic arch signal fluctuations in the arterial blood pressure via the glossopharyngeal and vagus nerves respectively. Similar receptors in the right atrium respond to central venous pressure. *Chemoreceptors* in the carotid bodies respond to reduced arterial oxygen, stimulating a brainstem inspiratory centre. Vagal bronchial afferents, activated progressively by stretch during inspiration, eventually inhibit this centre. Vagal afferents from the upper gastrointestinal tract mediate visceromotor, vasomotor and secretory reflexes. Sacral parasympathetic afferents convey awareness of vesical and lower colonic distension.

The gastrointestinal tract is insensitive to cutting and burning; pain results from the distension of hollow viscera, tension on mesenteries and compression of solid viscera. Impulses pass centrally via sympathetic afferents, but are often interpreted as 'referred pain', diffusely localized to the body surface with the same segmental innervation. Thus the early pain of appendicitis is referred to the periumbilical skin, since the midgut is median during development; if inflammation progresses, the parietal peritoneum (which has somatic innervation) is irritated and local pain occurs in the right iliac fossa. The heart is supplied by cervical and thoracic sympathetic branches, connecting with spinal segments T1–5; pain from coronary ischaemia (angina) is referred to the left side of the chest and lower neck and the inner surface of the left arm. Whereas the somatic muscle spasm which frequently accompanies visceral pain is a spinal reflex, referred pain is probably due to the thalamic proximity of equivalent somatic and visceral connexions.

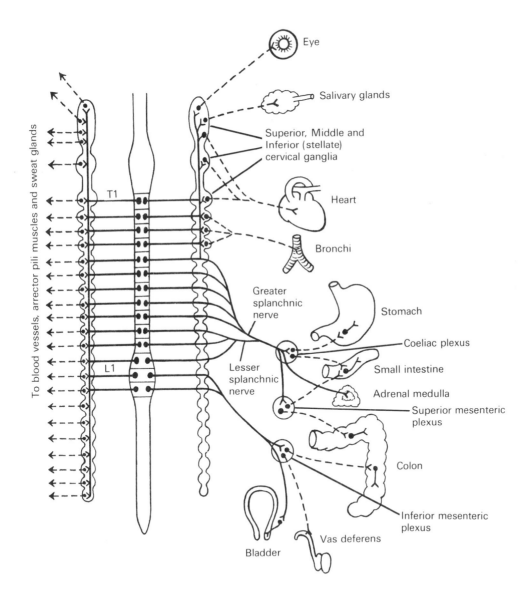

Fig. 3.9 Sympathetic nervous system. Postganglionic nerve fibres are indicated by interrupted lines.

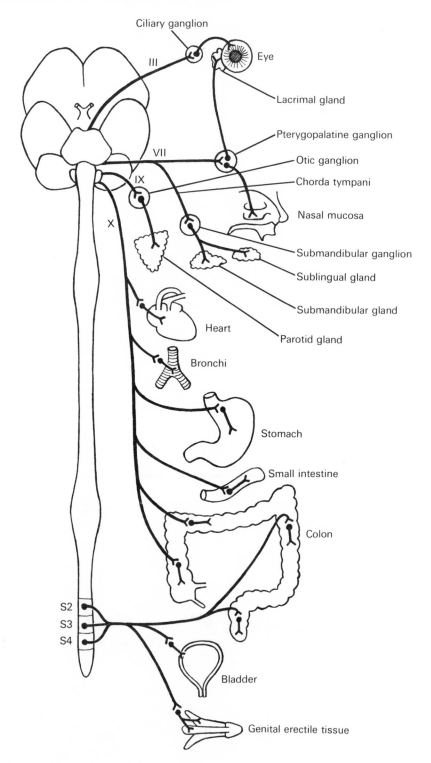

Fig. 3.10 Parasympathetic nervous system.

Visceral efferents

Preganglionic fibres (sympathetic and parasympathetic) are cholinergic. *Postganglionic* parasympathetic fibres are cholinergic, but sympathetic fibres are adrenergic except for the sudomotor fibres, which are cholinergic. Enteric innervation involves additional neurotransmitters and requires separate consideration (*see below*).

Sympathetic efferents leave via ventral roots (T1–L2), enter the spinal nerves, then form *white rami communicantes* (myelinated) to the ganglia of the sympathetic trunks which are paravertebral (*Fig.* 3.11). Having synapsed, some rejoin the spinal nerves by *grey rami communicantes* (non-myelinated) as vasomotor, sudomotor and pilomotor fibres. Some rostral efferents ascend in the sympathetic trunks and synapse in cervical ganglia, passing on to cervical nerves and, via the carotid plexuses, to cranial structures; similarly some caudal efferents descend to lumbar and sacral ganglia. Alternatively, efferents may *pass through* paravertebral ganglia to synapse in *prevertebral ganglia* (coeliac, superior and inferior mesenteric plexuses); a few terminate in the *suprarenal medulla*.

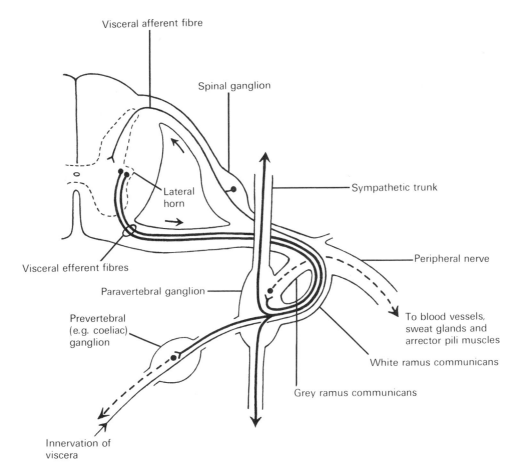

Fig. 3.11 Sympathetic efferent and afferent fibres. Postganglionic efferents are indicated by interrupted lines.

Parasympathetic outflow is via *cranial nerves* (oculomotor, facial, glossopharyngeal, vagus) and via the second to fourth *sacral nerves*, whose visceral efferents separate as *pelvic splanchnic nerves*. At cranial level preganglionic fibres synapse in the ciliary, pterygopalatine, submandibular and otic ganglia to supply the intrinsic ocular muscles, lacrimal and salivary glands. Postganglionic sympathetic efferents traverse but do not synapse in these ganglia. The vagus has a diffuse distribution to the thoracic and abdominal viscera but the pelvic organs and the terminal third of the colon are supplied by pelvic splanchnic nerves (*nervi erigentes*, being also motor to erectile tissue). The parasympathetic ganglia are close to the viscera, or in their walls; they form *cardiac and pulmonary plexuses*, an *intermuscular myenteric plexus (of Auerbach)* and *submucosal plexus (of Meissner)*. Pelvic splanchnic nerves join the pelvic sympathetic plexuses and synapse in minute ganglia; some ascend (in the sympathetic hypogastric plexus) to the descending and sigmoid colon.

Fibres leaving *autonomic ganglia* are more numerous than those entering, thus providing a dissemination of effect. Integration and processing also occurs by connexions between the principal cells and via interneurons (containing dopamine or noradrenaline) which form circuits between the afferent fibres and the principal cells. Parasympathetic effects are more discrete than sympathetic effects; there is less divergence and the action of the main parasympathetic neurotransmitter, acetylcholine, is quickly reversed by cholinesterase.

Enteric innervation

This has considerable anatomical and physiological independence from the central nervous system. Peristalsis is locally co-ordinated and is maintained even when central connexions are severed. The enteric ganglia are unusual; the submucosal plexus contains unipolar and bipolar primary afferent neurons. The myenteric plexus (between circular and longitudinal muscle layers) has features resembling the central nervous system: supporting cells like astrocytes surround all the neuronal elements; it is avascular; paraneuronal capillaries with tight intercellular junctions outside 'glia' resemble those in the brain. Postganglionic parasympathetic terminals are cholinergic; sympathetic terminals do not affect smooth muscle directly, but act by inhibiting parasympathetic fibres in ganglia. Numerous intrinsic neurons may contain either acetylcholine, 5–HT or substance P. Other neurotransmitters have been identified. Langley (1921) considered the 'enteric nervous system' unique and a third component of the autonomic system (in addition to sympathetic and parasympathetic). This subject attracts much research.

APPLIED ANATOMY

There are three main kinds of peripheral nerve injury. *Compression* results in *neurapraxia*, that is dysfunction without structural damage; temporary paralysis ensues, but there is rapid and total recovery. *Crushing* (axonotmesis) damages axons and myelin sheaths but endoneurial tubes are relatively intact, so full functional recovery is possible; after *severance* (neurotmesis) recovery is slower and usually incomplete, for reasons discussed above. Individual fasciculi can be reapposed by microsurgery. Sensory recovery follows a pattern: first there is the return of awareness of deep pressure, then of superficial pain poorly localized, followed by thermal sensation and, much later, light touch. Recovery of the most discriminative aspects of sensation is often imperfect, more so in proximal than in distal lesions. Amputation may be followed by continued, and sometimes painful, awareness of a *'phantom limb'*. Rarely, nerve injury is followed by continuous, intractable, disabling, burning pain (*causalgia*) and intense hyperaesthesia; it is imperfectly understood. One theory is that efferent sympathetic fibres artificially synapse with fine afferent (pain) fibres; sympathetic denervation is often curative.

A variety of conditions, nutritional (e.g. vitamin B deficiency), metabolic (e.g. diabetes mellitus), infective and toxic may cause *peripheral neuropathy*, resulting in negative phenomena due to loss of conduction and positive symptoms such as paraesthesiae ('pins and needles') due to spontaneous discharge.

The clinical relevance of retrograde axonal transport in rabies and tetanus is mentioned in Chapter 2. *Herpes zoster* ('shingles'), a viral infection of a spinal dorsal root ganglion or cranial sensory ganglion, causes pain in the corresponding dermatome, followed 24–48 hours later by a cutaneous blistering in the area, due to orthograde transport.

Occasionally clinical disorders directly affect neuromuscular transmission. *Botulism*, a fatal form of food poisoning, inhibits acetylcholine release at neuromuscular junctions. *Myasthenia gravis*, a rare state of weakness and fatigue in skeletal muscles, is due to an auto-immune reduction of acetylcholine receptors at neuromuscular junctions; it is alleviated by the anti-cholinesterase drug, neostigmine.

Local anaesthetics block axolemmal ionic exchange and affect non-myelinated and thinly myelinated (e.g. pain) fibres more rapidly and longer than thickly myelinated fibres.

Chapter 4

Spinal cord

GROSS ANATOMY

The spinal cord lies within the vertebral canal. In foetuses up to the age of 3 months, cord and canal are of equal length. Thereafter, the vertebral column grows more rapidly, so that at birth the caudal end of the cord is level with vertebra L3; in adults its caudal end is usually at the level of the first lumbar intervertebral disc (between L1 and L2). Cranially it continues into the medulla, just below the foramen magnum, its total length approximately 45 cm.

The cord is not of uniform diameter. It has two enlargements associated with the innervation of the limbs. The greatest diameter occurs at the *cervical enlargement* in cord

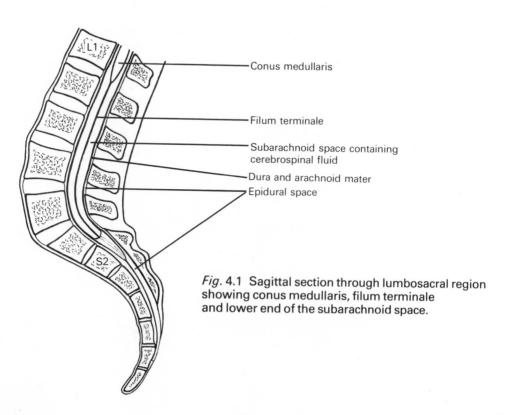

Conus medullaris

Filum terminale

Subarachnoid space containing cerebrospinal fluid

Dura and arachnoid mater

Epidural space

Fig. 4.1 Sagittal section through lumbosacral region showing conus medullaris, filum terminale and lower end of the subarachnoid space.

segments C4 to T1, concerned with the brachial plexus. The lumbar enlargement extends from cord segments L1 to S3. The caudal part of the cord forms the conical *conus medullaris*; from its tip, a fine thread of connective tissue, the *filum terminale*, extends to the dorsal side of the first piece of the coccyx (*Fig.* 4.1).

The spinal cord is enclosed in three layers, or *meninges*. The innermost *pia mater* adheres to the cord's surface. The *dura mater*, the outermost layer, is lined by the intermediate *arachnoid mater*, both these extending to the level of vertebra S2. The *subarachnoid space* between the pia and the arachnoid is filled by cerebrospinal fluid. To sample this, lumbar puncture can be safely carried out using a needle inserted in the midline between the third and fourth lumbar spines. The pia mater is drawn out on each side as *denticulate ligaments*, attached to the dura by twenty-one 'teeth'. An extradural or *epidural space* is occupied by adipose tissue and venous plexuses.

Each spinal cord segment gives origin to a pair of spinal nerves. There are 31 pairs of spinal nerves: 8 cervical, 12 thoracic, 5 lumbar, 5 sacral and 1 coccygeal. Since there are only seven cervical vertebrae, the first seven nerves pass cranial to the numerically corresponding neural arch but the eighth passes between C7 and T1. Caudal to this, each nerve occupies an intervertebral foramen caudal to the vertebra of the same number. Each pair of dorsal and ventral roots pierces the dura mater separately, the

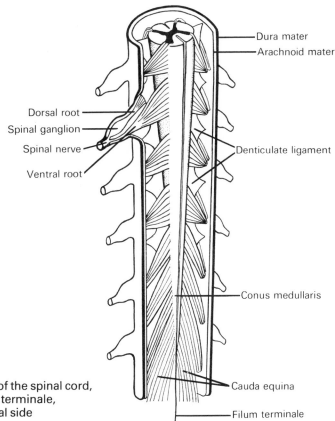

Fig. 4.2 The lower end of the spinal cord, cauda equina and filum terminale, exposed from the ventral side and viewed obliquely.

dura and epineurium fusing. Extradurally the roots traverse the epidural space and unite immediately distal to the dorsal root ganglion, within an intervertebral foramen.

Since an adult spinal cord is considerably shorter than its vertebral column, some nerve roots pass obliquely from the cord, this obliquity increasing caudally. The lumbar, sacral and coccygeal roots together form a leash, the *cauda equina*, around the filum terminale (*Fig.* 4.2). Spinal cord segments are generally situated cranial to the numerically equivalent vertebrae. Thus segment T1 is opposite vertebra C7, L1 is opposite T11, sacral and coccygeal segments are posterior to vertebra L1.

A *ventral median fissure* throughout the whole ventral aspect is partly filled by a thickening of the pia, the *linea splendens*, and contains the anterior spinal artery. Deep to it is the anterior white commissure. From a shallow *dorsal median sulcus*, a midline neuroglial septum extends to the grey commissure.

GREY MATTER AND NUCLEI

The grey matter has a variable butterfly profile (*Fig.* 4.3). The grey commissure encloses a small central canal. On each side there are dorsal and ventral grey columns, referred to in sections as 'horns'. The intermediate area has a small lateral horn in segments T1–L2. The amount of grey matter is increased in the cervical and lumbar enlargements. The cord segments are not of equal length: lumbar and sacral segments are relatively short, increasing the area of grey matter seen in sections at these levels.

'Nuclei' are aggregations of nerve cell bodies, usually with common functions and on a common pathway. In the following description, these extend throughout the cord (*Figs.* 4.4, 4.5) unless otherwise stated.

Dorsal horn (somatic and visceral afferent)

1. *Substantia gelatinosa.* This caps the apex of the dorsal horn, and contains small Golgi Type II neurons and fine fibres. It modulates afferent patterns in respect of pain perception. At its tip is a small posterior marginal nucleus.
2. *Nucleus proprius.* Forming most of the dorsal horn, this contains bodies of secondary sensory neurons subserving pain, temperature and touch.
3. *Thoracic nucleus* (nucleus dorsalis of Clarke). Extending through T1 to L2, this is the location of the bodies of secondary sensory neurons carrying proprioceptive impulses to the cerebellum and is situated medial to the base of the dorsal horn. An ascending input enlarges the caudal end of Clarke's column, which also has, at its cranial end, a descending input from the lower cervical region. Proprioceptive afferents from the upper cervical spinal nerves ascend to the medulla (accessory cuneate nucleus).
4. *Visceral afferent nucleus.* This extends from T1 to L2 (sympathetic), and from S2 to S4 (parasympathetic), and is sited laterally in the base of the dorsal horn. It receives visceral afferents from nerve cells in the dorsal root ganglia.

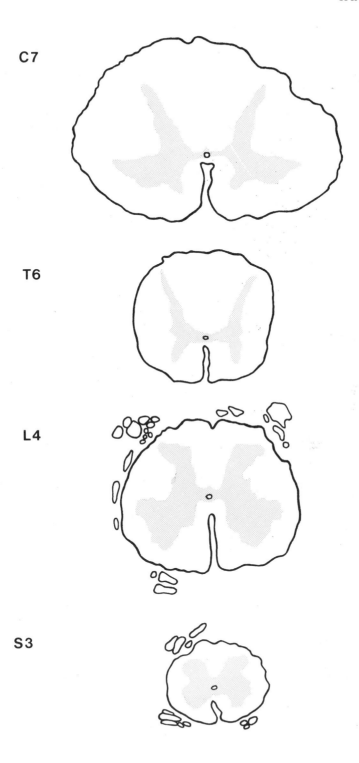

C7

T6

L4

S3

Fig. 4.3 Transverse sections of the spinal cord to indicate general profiles and relative amounts of white and grey matter in various segments.

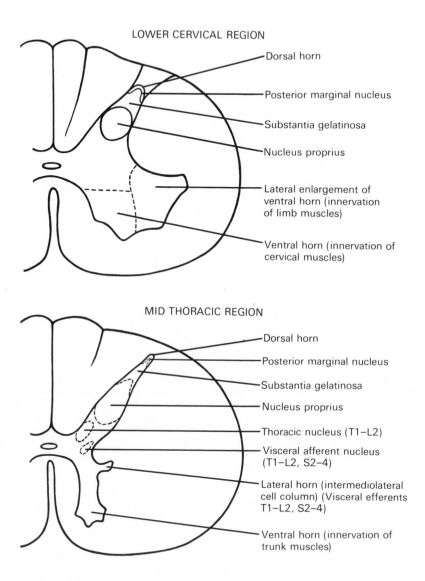

LOWER CERVICAL REGION

— Dorsal horn

— Posterior marginal nucleus

— Substantia gelatinosa

— Nucleus proprius

— Lateral enlargement of ventral horn (innervation of limb muscles)

— Ventral horn (innervation of cervical muscles)

MID THORACIC REGION

— Dorsal horn

— Posterior marginal nucleus

— Substantia gelatinosa

— Nucleus proprius

— Thoracic nucleus (T1–L2)

— Visceral afferent nucleus (T1–L2, S2–4)

— Lateral horn (intermediolateral cell column) (Visceral efferents T1–L2, S2–4)

— Ventral horn (innervation of trunk muscles)

Fig. 4.4 Grey matter of the spinal cord.

Lateral horn (visceral efferent)

The cell bodies of preganglionic sympathetic efferent neurons occupy the inter-mediolateral cell column (T1–L2), a characteristic feature of thoracic sections. The nucleus of origin of the sacral parasympathetic outflow (S2–S4) is nearer to the central canal.

Ventral horn (somatic efferent)

Many descending pathways, sometimes referred to as 'upper motor neurons', converge on ventral horn cells, the lower motor neurons which form the 'final common pathway'. There are two cell types: large α motor neurons innervating extrafusal muscle fibres and smaller γ motor neurons supplying intrafusal muscle fibres of the neuromuscular spindles.

A medial column, extending throughout all levels, supplies trunk and neck musculature. The cervical and lumbar enlargements are identified by lateral extensions of the ventral horn, in which functional groups supplying muscles with a common effect on a joint, such as flexion or extension, can be recognized.

A *central nucleus* in cord segments C3, C4 and C5 is the origin of the phrenic nerve. A similar central lumbosacral nucleus has an uncertain distribution. The spinal accessory nerve, unique in emerging by a row of rootlets from the lateral aspect of the cord, ascends via the foramen magnum. It originates from an *accessory nucleus*, dorsolateral in the ventral horn of the upper five or six cervical segments. it supplies muscles of branchial arch origin, hence its unusual features.

The laminar architecture of Rexed

As might be expected, the organization of spinal grey matter is much more complex than is evident from the study of large nuclei at low magnification. Detailed investi-gation of cytoarchitecture, experimental examination of the effects of cutting posterior nerve roots and supraspinal paths, and electrophysiological recordings have revealed a laminar functional pattern of cells: ten laminae, as described by Rexed in cats, and shown in *Fig.* 4.6, are briefly described here.

Laminae I–IV, near the apex of dorsal horn, are receptive zones for cutaneous afferents. Each layer has identifiable cell patterns and synaptic fields. Laminae V and VI are at the base of the dorsal horn. Lamina V receives input from superficial laminae in addition to primary afferents; efferent fibres form contralateral spinothalamic tracts. Lamina VI is only prominent in cord segments associated with the limbs and appears to receive proprioceptive impulses: microelectrode studies show that only these cells respond to movement. Lamina VII is the intermediate zone between the dorsal and ventral horns, including the thoracic nucleus, visceral afferent and efferent nuclei and many interneurons. Lamina IX largely consists of α and γ motor neurons whose dendritic fields extend into lamina VII. Lamina X is part of the grey commissure.

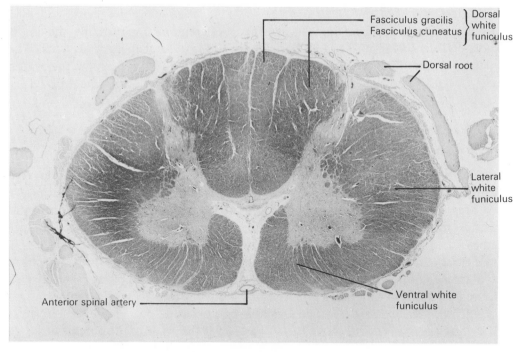

Fasciculus gracilis ⎫ Dorsal
Fasciculus cuneatus ⎬ white
                    ⎭ funiculus

Dorsal root

Lateral white funiculus

Ventral white funiculus

Anterior spinal artery

A

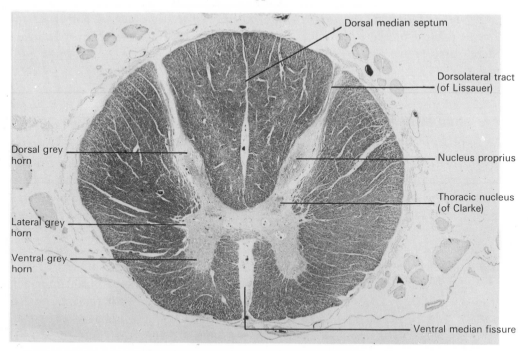

Dorsal median septum

Dorsolateral tract (of Lissauer)

Dorsal grey horn

Nucleus proprius

Thoracic nucleus (of Clarke)

Lateral grey horn

Ventral grey horn

Ventral median fissure

B

Fig. 4.5 (A) Transverse section of lower cervical cord (Weigert stain, × 8.) (B) Transverse section of midthoracic cord. (Weigert stain, × 10.) (C) Transverse section of lumbar cord. (Weigert stain, × 8.) (D) Transverse section of sacral cord. (Weigert stain, × 12.)

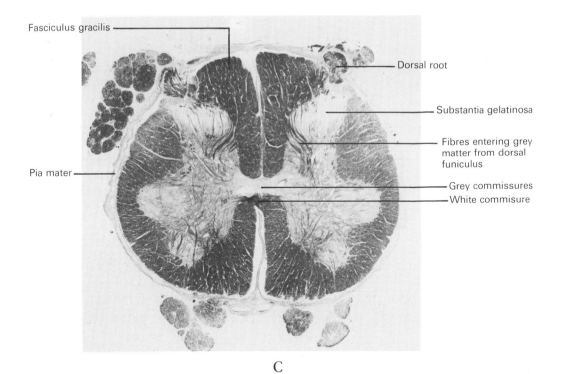

Fasciculus gracilis

Dorsal root

Substantia gelatinosa

Fibres entering grey matter from dorsal funiculus

Pia mater

Grey commissures
White commisure

C

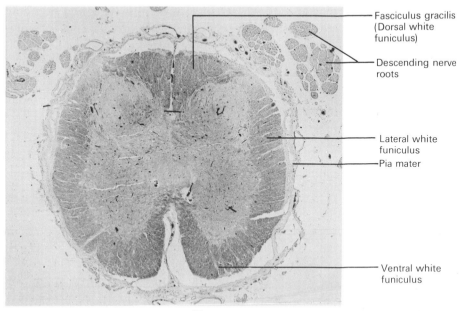

Fasciculus gracilis (Dorsal white funiculus)

Descending nerve roots

Lateral white funiculus
Pia mater

Ventral white funiculus

D

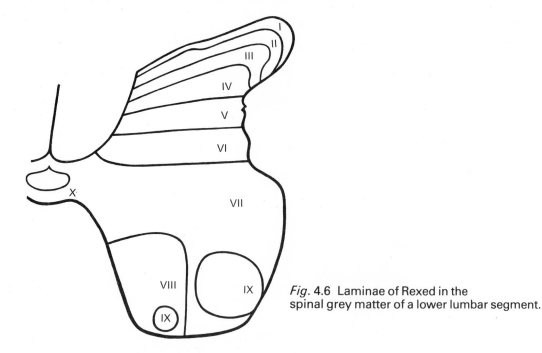

Fig. 4.6 Laminae of Rexed in the spinal grey matter of a lower lumbar segment.

Corticospinal fibres from 'sensory' cortical areas terminate in laminae IV and V and, with descending fibres from the brainstem, influence sensory input. In cats, cortico-spinal fibres from the 'motor' cortex terminate on interneurons in laminae V–VII. In primates some corticospinal fibres synapse directly with α and γ motor neurons. Reticulospinal and vestibulospinal fibres synapse with interneurons in laminae VII and VIII.

Spinal cord nuclei and corresponding laminae:

Nuclei	*Laminae*	*Regions*
Posterior marginal nucleus	I	Dorsal horn
Substantia gelatinosa	II, III	Dorsal horn
Nucleus proprius	IV, V	Dorsal horn
Thoracic nucleus (T1–L2)	VII	Intermediate zone
Visceral nuclei (T1–L2, S2–4)	VII	Intermediate zone
Somatomotor nuclei	IX	Ventral horn

INTRINSIC SPINAL MECHANISMS

Between the dorsal and ventral horns are many small cells with short axons known as *internuncial neurons*, or interneurons, commonly interposed between descending fibres and ventral horn cells. Some are inhibitory, for example when a 'prime mover' is stimulated, its antagonist must synchronously be inhibited. *Association neurons* are restricted to one side (ipsilateral), while axons of *commissural neurons* cross the midline. An interneuron may be limited to one segment, or it may be intersegmental (plurisegmental).

A *reflex arc* requires: (1) a sensory receptor, (2) a sensory neuron = afferent pathway, (3) a central synapse, sometimes via interneurons, (4) a motor neuron = efferent pathway, (5) an effector, for example muscle fibres, glands, etc.

In *flexor reflex* (*Fig.* 4.7A) a limb is withdrawn in reaction to painful cutaneous stimulus. Its path is polysynaptic and its response clearly involves several segments.

A *stretch reflex* (*Fig.* 4.7B) is monosynaptic and exemplified by tapping a patellar tendon. When a muscle is stretched, receptors in its neuromuscular spindles respond; afferent impulses then cause spinal α motor neurons to fire and the skeletal muscle contracts. Such reflexes counteract stretch and are involved in maintaining posture.

Neuromuscular spindle (intrafusal) receptors are stimulated by passive stretch or active contraction of intrafusal muscle.

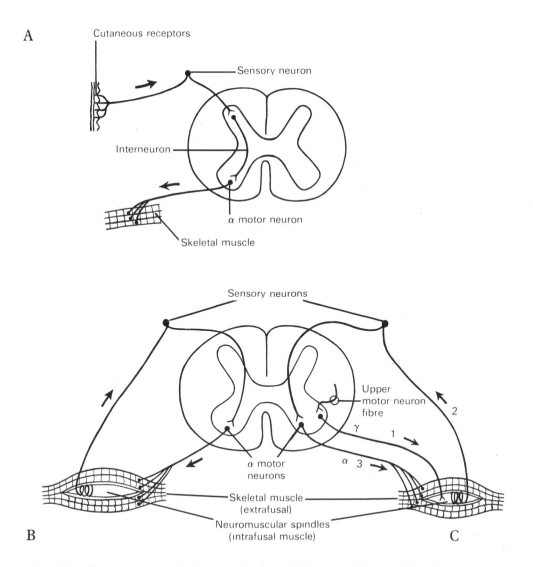

Fig. 4.7 Spinal reflex arcs. (A) Flexor reflex arc. (B) Stretch reflex arc. (C) γ reflex loop.

In the so-called γ *reflex loop* (*Fig.* 4.7C) upper motor neurons at cranial level activate γ motor neurons in the ventral horn, causing intrafusal muscle to contract. This stimulates intrafusal receptors and, via the stretch reflex efferents, α motor neurons fire to make skeletal muscle contract. Since the spindles are attached at their ends to skeletal muscle connective tissue, the shortening of skeletal muscle reduces tension in the spindles and the rates of afferent discharge diminish. This servo-type system enables surrounding skeletal muscle to adjust in relation to the predetermined length of the spindle.

WHITE MATTER AND TRACTS

The white matter of the cord (*Fig.* 4.8) is in three columns or *funiculi*. The *ventral funiculus* is between the ventral median fissure and the ventral spinal roots, the *lateral funiculus* between the dorsal and ventral roots, and *dorsal funiculus* between the dorsal spinal roots and dorsal median septum. The two dorsal funiculi are often named *dorsal columns*. The absolute amount of spinal white matter increases cranially, ascending tracts enlarging upwards, descending tracts progressively reducing as they descend. The cord diameter is greatest in the lower cervical region.

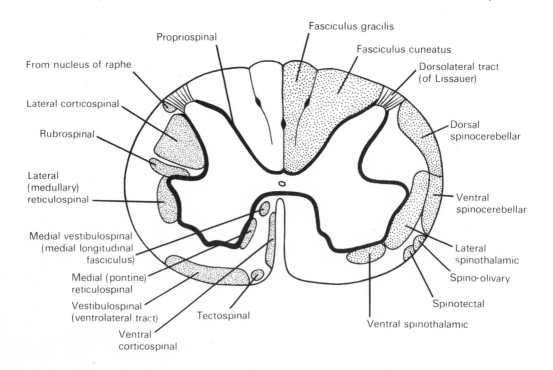

Fig. 4.8 A simplified diagram of the main tracts of the spinal cord. Ascending tracts are on the right, descending tracts on the left. Propriospinal tracts are shown in black.

Ascending tracts

Pathways to the cerebral cortex via the thalamus

Tracts ascending to the contralateral cerebral cortex are in three-neuron chains: the primary neurons have bodies in dorsal root ganglia, the tertiary are thalamic and the secondary (intermediate) are in the spinal dorsal grey matter or the dorsal medulla. Tracts in the dorsal half of the cord are uncrossed, but ventral fibres have crossed the midline.

Dorsal root fibres enter the cord as two groups; heavily myelinated fibres form a *medial division*, entering the dorsal columns and conveying impulses concerned in proprioception, vibration, touch and pressure, while non-myelinated and thinly myelinated fibres form a *lateral division*, concerned in pain and temperature modalities.

PAIN AND TEMPERATURE PATHWAYS

Fine fibres enter the *dorsolateral tract* (of Lissauer), ascending or descending a segment before entering the dorsal horn; all end in the substantia gelatinosa. Their secondary neurons are in the *nucleus proprius*, with dendrites extending into the substantia gelatinosa to synapse with incoming fibres either directly or via interneurons. Axons from the nucleus proprius cross in the anterior white and grey commissures to form a *lateral spinothalamic tract*; of recent evolution, this tract contains only 1 500–2 000 fibres even in man. Alternative *spinoreticular* pain pathways involve the reticular formation, a diffuse, phylogenetically ancient bilateral network of polysynaptic fibres, ascending and descending throughout the cord and brainstem. Visceral pain is mediated by both pathways: hence surgical division of the lateral spinothalamic tract may only partly relieve intractable pain. Dorsal root autonomic afferents synapse with neurons of the visceral afferent nucleus at the base of the dorsal horn.

General sensory afferents from the face are in the trigeminal nerve, primary sensory neurons in its ganglion, the secondary neurons in the trigeminal sensory nucleus of the brainstem and upper cervical cord. From this nucleus *trigeminothalamic tracts* arise. (Trigeminal nuclei and tracts are described in Chapter 6). Pain pathways are illustrated in *Fig.* 4.9.

PAIN RESEARCH

Increased understanding of pain has accrued in recent years. In 1965 Melzack and Wall proposed the gate control theory of pain. In 1969 Reynolds showed that stimulation of mesencephalic central grey matter produces deep analgesia without loss of consciousness. In 1974 Pert, Snowman and Snyder localized endogenous opiate-like substances, enkephalins and endorphins, in synaptic membranes and their release was later shown to be associated with pain relief.

PAIN PERCEPTION

All perception is complex and largely still under investigation. Individuals vary in their 'pain threshold'; anticipation and fear lower it, and increase the perceived intensity of pain. A soldier may sustain a grievous wound but, in the heat of battle, be unaware of it. *Central inhibition* of pain pathways may occur at central nervous levels. There is also

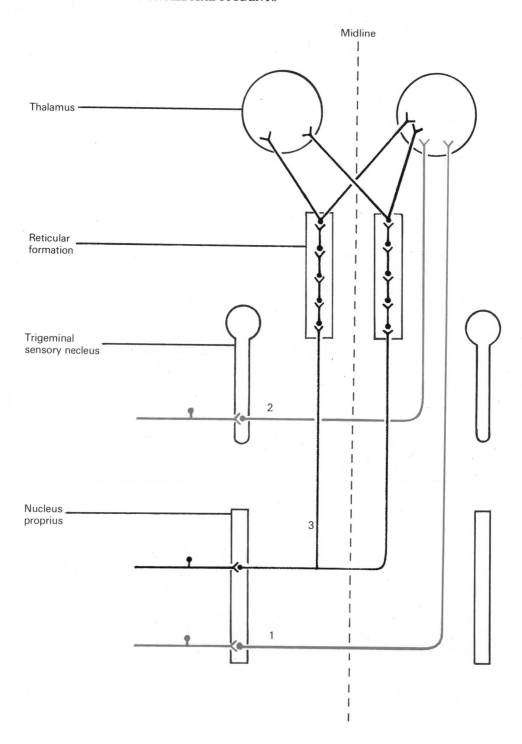

Fig. 4.9 Diagram of pain pathways. 1: Lateral spinothalamic tract. 2: Trigeminothalamic tract. 3: Bilateral spinoreticular pathways. (Adapted from Sinclair D. C. (1967) *Cutaneous Sensation*. Oxford, Oxford University Press.)

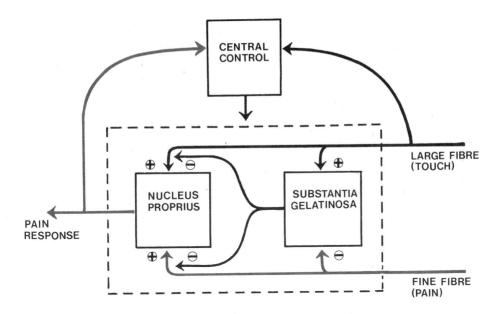

Fig. 4.10 Schematic diagram of the theoretical gate control mechanism in the perception of and response to painful stimuli. Note excitation (+) and inhibition (−). (Adapted from Melzack R. and Wall P. D. (1965) *Science*, **150**, 971.)

evidence of *peripheral inhibition* of pain transmission (e.g. rubbing a bumped elbow appears to relieve the pain). An explanation of inhibition in nociceptor (pain) transmission was proposed in the 'gate theory' (*Fig.* 4.10). In simple terms, such transmission is affected by competition between large and small fibre input to inhibitory interneurons in the substantia gelatinosa; large (tactile) fibres stimulate these intrinsic cells; small 'pain fibres' de-activate their inhibitory effect on afferents to the nucleus proprius. This dorsal horn complex receives collaterals from descending corticospinal fibres, providing a path to override sensory input under certain circumstances. In its original form this theory was not experimentally verifiable, and has now been modified. Nevertheless its clinical predictions proved valuable: electrical or mechanical stimulation of sensory nerves may sometimes provide relief of intractable pain.

A signal advance in concepts of pain mechanisms has been the identification of opiate receptors in several regions of the central grey matter. In the spinal cord, receptors and enkephalin occur in the substantia gelatinosa and act as pain suppressors (*Fig.* 4.11). Cells in the periaqueductal mesencephalic grey matter and medullary raphé nucleus can be activated by collaterals from ascending or descending pathways. Fibres from the brainstem in the dorsolateral tract to dorsal horn interneurons release enkephalin which, in turn, causes presynaptic inhibition in the pain pathway. A peptide, substance P, appears in the central terminals of pain fibres (AIII and C), probably as a primary transmitter in the pathway. Substance P is not present in dorsal column nuclei.

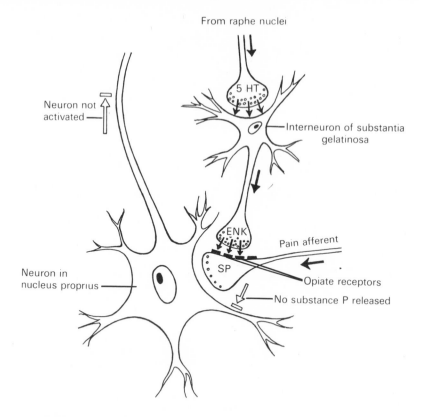

Fig. 4.11 Enkephalin-mediated pain suppression. Raphé nuclei of the brainstem (which produce the neurotransmitter serotonin, **5–HT**) synapse by descending fibres in the dorsolateral spinal tract with interneurons of the substantia gelatinosa (containing enkephalin, **ENK**). Enkephalin binds to opiate receptors of the afferent pain terminals, blocking the release of substance P, (**SP**); neurons in the nucleus proprius are not activated. (Adapted from Ottoson D. (1983) *Physiology of the Nervous System.* London, Macmillan.)

SIMPLE TOUCH AND PRESSURE (*Fig.* 4.12)

Dorsal root fibres concerned in these modalities are large and myelinated, entering the cord by the roots' medial divisions to the dorsal columns, where they bifurcate into short descending and longer ascending fibres, which end in the dorsal grey zone in six to eight segments. There is thus a marked overlap of central input from adjacent dorsal roots. Secondary fibres, arising in the *nucleus proprius*, cross to form a contralateral *ventral spinothalamic tract*. Finer tactile and spatial discriminations are not served by this pathway.

DISCRIMINATIVE TOUCH, CONSCIOUS PROPRIOCEPTION, VIBRATION (*Fig.* 4.12)

The dorsal columns convey long (ipsilateral) projection fibres for the above modalites, extending from the dorsal root ganglia to the medulla. They also carry 'passenger' fibres which ascend or descend before entering the dorsal horn nuclei or, in some spinal

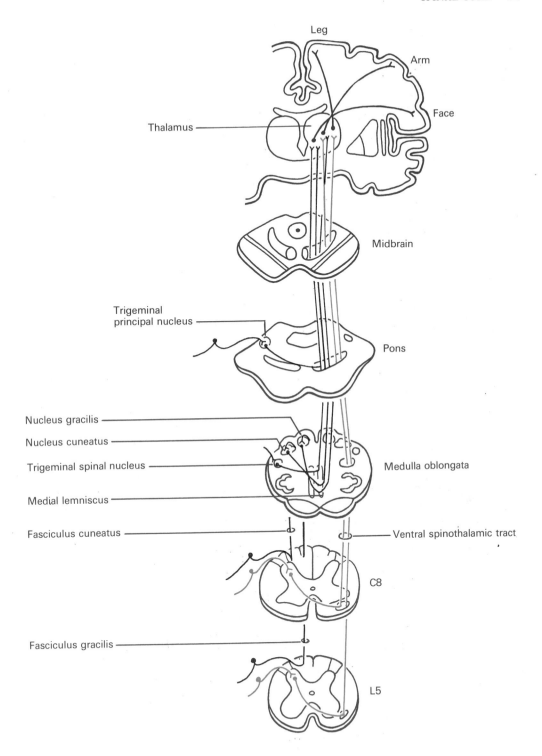

Fig. 4.12 Ascending pathways for tactile sensation. The dorsal column-medial lemniscal path is in blue, the ventral spinothalamic tract is in red.

reflexes, synapsing with ventral motor neurons. Long ascending fibres form a *dorsal column-medial lemniscal pathway*. Fibres entering below midthoracic level accumulate medially to form the *fasciculus gracilis*; the input above this is to the *fasciculus cuneatus*. Cell bodies of secondary neurons are in the *nuclei gracilis and cuneatus*, located dorsally in the lower medulla. The pathway then crosses in the *sensory decussation* to form the *medial lemniscus*, which ascends through the brainstem to the thalamus ('lemniscus' means a ribbon or fillet). It also receives a trigeminothalamic input as it ascends.

The pathway is a highly discriminative one, both spatially and in the specificity of fibres for each modality, ensured by relatively discrete synapses, limited divergence, and by 'surround inhibition'. Dorsal column integrity may be tested clinically to illustrate these features. If a subject's finger or toe is moved by an examiner, the individual can state, with closed eyes, which digit is being moved, and in what direction (conscious proprioception or kinaesthesia). Spatial touch is tested by 'two-point discrimination'. These abilities are also apparent in handling familiar objects. Vibration (rapidly repeated signals of short duration) is tested by applying a tuning fork to bony prominences such as the medial malleolus.

As noted above, the lower half of the body is represented medially in the dorsal columns, the upper half laterally, since fibres feed into the pathway from the lateral aspect. In crossed spinothalamic tracts, input is from the medial aspect, and somatic representation is reversed. Since both paths project to the same thalamic region, somatic orientation must be aligned in the brainstem; this occurs in the medial lemniscal pathway. The sensory decussation involves one 90° rotation, and a further 90° rotation occurs as the medial lemniscus ascends (*Fig.* 4.12).

Pathways to the cerebellum

In contrast to cerebral tracts, those leading to the cerebellum provide an *ipsilateral input*, and form a two-neuron chain.

DORSAL SPINOCEREBELLAR TRACT

The cell bodies of primary neurons are in dorsal root ganglia, those of secondary neurons in the *thoracic nucleus* (nucleus dorsalis): since this nucleus occurs only in cord segments T1–L2, input fibres from below L2 must ascend in the dorsal columns before entering the grey matter. The nucleus is therefore large at its caudal end; fibres also descend from cervical spinal nerves C5–C8 to its upper part. Axons from the ipsilateral thoracic nucleus form a dorsal spinocerebellar tract ascending to the cerebellum via its inferior peduncle.

CUNEOCEREBELLAR TRACT

Proprioceptive input from spinal nerves C1–C4 passes to the *accessory cuneate nucleus*, on the medulla's dorsal aspect, and thence to the inferior cerebellar peduncle. It should be noted that the *accessory cuneate* and the cuneate (i.e. the dorsal column-lemniscal) nuclei, though adjacent, are on different pathways and subserve different functions.

VENTRAL SPINOCEREBELLAR TRACT

This tract transmits impulses only from the hind limb and lower trunk. The exact location of its secondary neuron bodies is uncertain. It has ipsilateral and contralateral fibres, the latter re-crossing at cerebellar level, so that the ultimate input to the cerebellum is all ipsilateral. It enters the cerebellum via the superior peduncle.

Other tracts

INDIRECT SPINOCEREBELLAR PATHS

The spino-olivary tract is small, and ends in the inferior olive, a folded grey mass in the medulla. Most of the olivary input comes from higher centres. The inferior olive projects to the cerebellum via the inferior peduncle.

Spinoreticular fibres provide a path to the medullary reticular formation which sends efferents to the cerebellum via its inferior peduncle.

SPINOTECTAL TRACT

This small crossed tract, most distinct at cervical cord level, is a supplementary pain pathway ending in the superior colliculus, part of the midbrain roof or tectum. Reflex head movements in response to visual or auditory stimuli are mediated via the tectum: the spinotectal tract is concerned with similar reactions to pain.

PROPRIOSPINAL TRACTS

The *fasciculus proprius* consists of ascending and descending association fibres immediately peripheral to the grey matter, and probably mediates intersegmental reflexes. Some long polysynaptic reticular paths in the lateral funiculus are in this junctional zone.

Descending tracts (*Fig.* 4.8)

Descending motor control pathways are often grouped as *pyramidal* and *extrapyramidal*. The pyramidal tract extends from the cerebral cortex to ventral horn cells of the spinal cord (corticospinal) and to some cranial nerve nuclei (corticobulbar). The extra-pyramidal 'system' includes all other motor tracts. The pyramidal tract, relatively recently evolved, is superimposed upon a phylogenetically more ancient and diverse pattern (*Fig.* 4.13). In lower vertebrates the somatomotor and visceromotor 'control centres' (corpus striatum and hypothalamus) operate through the polysynaptic *reticulospinal* path. Equilibration control is via the archecerebellum and vestibular nuclei to the *vestibulospinal* tract. The tectum, important in visual and auditory motor reflexes, has its *tectospinal* tract. In the primate pattern, the highly developed cerebral cortex has its own direct path, and also acts via some extrapyramidal nuclei (e.g. red nucleus). However, in man the corpus striatum influences descending pathways principally via its cortical connexions. The two systems are anatomically and physio-logically interlocked, and both are usually included in the clinical term 'upper motor neuron lesion'.

The pyramidal system

This is so named because the corticospinal tract traverses the medullary pyramids, but it also includes corticobulbar fibres descending to the brainstem motor nuclei of cranial nerves (*Fig.* 4.14).

The primary motor cortex, anterior to the central sulcus, is the source of 40% of the pyramidal fibres; the remainder arise in the premotor area of the frontal lobe and from the parietal cortex. The neuronal somata are pyramidal, and 3% are so-called 'giant pyramidal' or Betz cells.

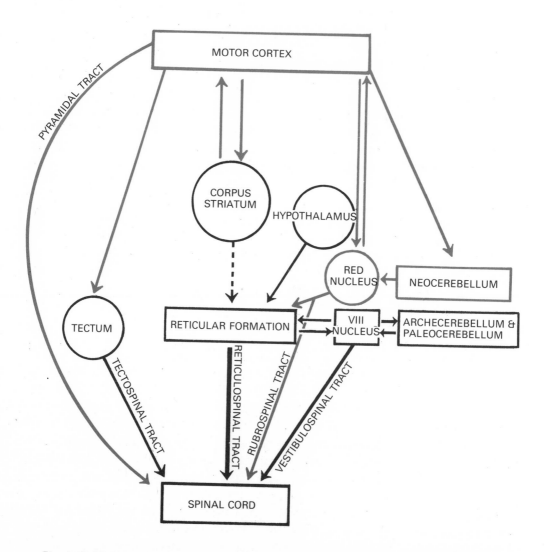

Fig. 4.13 Motor pathways. Advanced features (in red) present in a primate are superimposed on a lower vertebrate system (in black). The human corpus striatum influences descending tracts principally via its cortical connexions; a projection to the mesencephalic reticular formation is shown by an interrupted line.

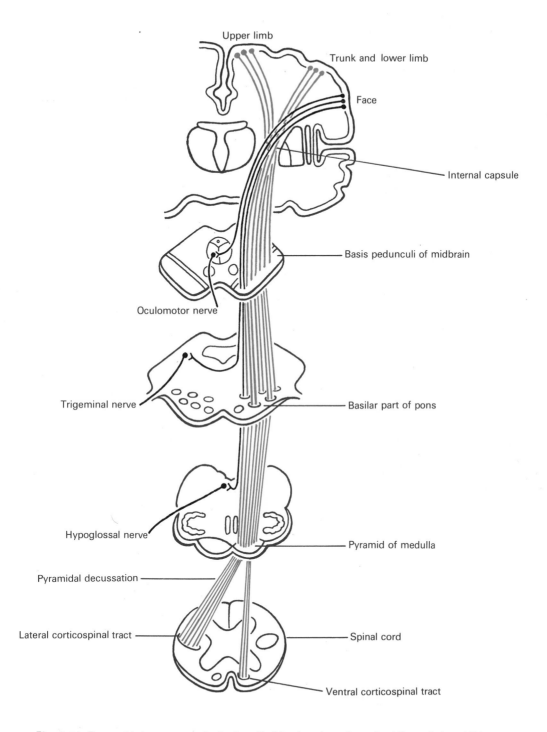

Fig. 4.14 Pyramidal tracts, corticobulbar (in blue) and corticospinal (in red). In addition to the cranial nerves shown, corticobulbar fibres innervate the motor nuclei of the trochlear, abducent and facial nerves and the nucleus ambiguus (of the glosso-pharyngeal, vagus and cranial accessory nerves).

Cortical motor representation of the body is such that the lower limbs are supero-medial and the face inferolateral. Moreover, the areas of motor cortex innervating individual parts are related to functional motor significance and innervation density, rather than to size; thus neurons to the face, tongue, larynx and hand occupy large areas.

The pyramidal tract, of about a million fibres, descends through the posterior limb of the internal capsule, occupies the middle three-fifths of the basis pedunculi in the mid-brain, separates into bundles in the pons, and forms the pyramid on the ventromedial medullary aspect, where the two tracts are adjacent, flanking the midline. In the lower medulla 85% of the fibres pass in the *pyramidal decussation* to form a *lateral corticospinal tract* in each lateral funiculus. The remainder continue into the ipsilateral ventral funiculus as a *ventral corticospinal tract*, descending to the cervical and upper thoracic regions. Many ventral tract fibres in fact cross in the cord prior to termination: *the corticospinal projection thus is essentially contralateral*, that is the left cerebral hemisphere controls the right side of the body. A small number of fibres from the pyramid continue ipsilaterally either into the lateral tract, or as uncrossed ventral tract fibres. Corticospinal fibres connect, mostly via interneurons, with α motor neurons and some γ motor neurons of the ventral grey column, 50% terminating in cervical segments, 20% in thoracic segments, 30% in lumbosacral segments.

As the pyramidal tract traverses the brainstem, corticobulbar fibres supply motor nuclei of the cranial nerves. Some cross the midline, others do not. Some cranial nerve nuclei may receive a bilateral cortical innervation.

The principal feature of corticospinal tracts is that axons descend from their cortical origins to their spinal terminations without interruption. Extrapyramidal tracts have intermediate synapses in their courses.

A corticospinal tract gives off collaterals as it descends, some passing to extra-pyramidal nuclei, interlocking the two systems. Other branches, passing to secondary sensory neurons such as the nucleus proprius or the cuneate and gracile nuclei, influence the central transmission of sensory impulses.

The extrapyramidal system

VESTIBULOSPINAL TRACTS

These, originating in the vestibular nuclei, which receive afferents via the eighth cranial nerve from the aural labyrinth, have intimate cerebellar connexions. A large *ventro-lateral vestibulospinal tract* starts in the lateral vestibular (Deiter's) nucleus and descends uncrossed throughout the cord. It facilitates extensor musculature in the anti-gravity maintenance of posture. A smaller *medial vestibulospinal tract* begins in the medial vestibular nucleus and descends, crossed and uncrossed, to cervical segments. It conveys vestibular influences to the neck and forelimb muscles, and is continued rostrally throughout the brainstem as an association fasciculus, the *medial longitudinal fasciculus*.

RETICULOSPINAL TRACTS

The reticular formation extends throughout the brainstem as a phylogenetically primitive reticulum or network of small neurons. It has a diverse input, but its descending connexions are mostly from the cerebral cortex, extrapyramidal nuclei and cerebellum, and it is thus concerned with muscle tone through muscle spindle control. There are inhibitory and excitatory zones in the reticular formation. The tracts are not well localized in the spinal cord and contain long and short polysynaptic routes. The *lateral reticulospinal tract* is deep in the lateral funiculus, mingling with the fasciculus proprius. It starts in the medullary reticular formation and has a bilateral inhibitory effect. The smaller *medial reticulospinal tract* consists of fibres scattered in the anterior funiculus which descend ipsilaterally from the pontine reticular formation and are facilitatory.

RUBROSPINAL TRACT
The red nuclei, two large mesencephalic masses flanking the midline, receive cerebellar afferents and project to the reticular formation; some descending fibres decussate in the midbrain to form the rubrospinal tract in the lateral funiculus of the cord. The tract enhances flexor muscle activity in limbs during locomotion.

TECTOSPINAL TRACT
This arises in the superior colliculus of the midbrain tectum. Its fibres decussate at once and descend to cervical level. The tract is involved in reflex head movements in response to visual, auditory and painful stimuli.

Functional comparison of pyramidal and extrapyramidal systems

Extrapyramidal tracts are concerned with locomotion, posture, trunk and head movements. Experimental transection of the medullary pyramids abolishes discrete movements of the hands, fingers, feet and toes. Corticospinal tracts are essential to skilled movements, but extrapyramidal fibres 'set the stage' by holding the limbs in required positions. The two systems are interlocked and, with the cerebellum, are involved in the co-ordination of muscles (synergy) and the regulation of muscle tone.

Descending autonomic fibres

Visceromotor fibres descend from the hypothalamus, and from regulatory cardio-vascular and respiratory centres in the medulla and pons via a polysynaptic visceral efferent pathway, interspersed with other reticulospinal fibres in the lateral funiculus. Its multisynaptic nature makes localization experimentally difficult.

APPLIED ANATOMY

SENSORY ATAXIA. Ataxia is inco-ordination of movement and occurs in diseases of the cerebellum (cerebellar ataxia), or damage to the dorsal spinal columns (sensory ataxia). The spinal cord diameter is greatest in the lower cervical region, a very mobile part of the vertebral column. Collagenous degeneration causes ligamenta flava to deform and buckle when the neck extends: *cervical compression* of the dorsal columns ensues.

Subacute combined degeneration of the cord is caused by vitamin B_{12} deficiency. Ataxia and paraesthesia are symptoms of dorsal column demyelination. The term 'combined' is used because motor pathways are also affected. *Tabes dorsalis* (locomotor ataxia), an advanced form of syphilis, causes atrophy of the dorsal columns and also affects dorsal spinal roots, leading to proprioceptive and general sensory loss.

PAIN PATHWAYS. *Syringomyelia* is congenital cystic cavitation of the central canal, which destroys commissural fibres of the spinothalamic tracts. 'Dissociated anaesthesia' ensues: loss of pain sensation, with tactile paths in dorsal columns unaffected.

Referred pain is pain from a visceral source referred to an area of the body surface with the same segmental innervation. Thus the early pain in appendicitis is referred to the peri-umbilical region. Spinal and supraspinal paths are involved.

The Brown-Séquard syndrome follows spinal hemisection. Pain and temperature sensation are lost contralateral to the lesion. Touch sensation is little affected because it has both ipsilateral (dorsal column) and contralateral (ventral spinothalamic) paths. There is also ipsilateral motor loss.

MOTOR PATHWAYS. Transection of the spinal cord at level C4 results in loss of diaphragmatic and intercostal muscle action, with respiratory paralysis. A lesion between C4 and T1 paralyses all four limbs (quadriplegia), the severity of paralysis in the upper limbs depending on the level of section. Damage to segment T1 affects small muscles in the hands. Section at T1 or above interrupts the sympathetic efferent pathway, and its outflow at this level to the head. Signs of sympathetic denervation of the head are included in *Horner's syndrome:* on the side of lesion there is pupillary constriction (miosis), loss of sweating of the face (anhydrosis), drooping of upper eyelid (ptosis; levator palpebrae superioris contains some smooth muscle), and apparent enophthalmos. Damage at midthoracic level results in paralysis of the lower limbs (paraplegia). Section at S1 causes loss of sacral parasympathetic control over the bladder and rectum.

An *upper motor neuron lesion* almost always involves pyramidal *and* extrapyramidal tracts, causing spasticity and exaggerated tendon reflexes, but little atrophy of affected muscles ensues. Stretch reflex arcs are still intact but have lost supraspinal control.

If ventral horn cells are destroyed, as in poliomyelitis, or peripheral nerves are damaged, a *lower motor neuron lesion* results. There is severe atrophy of muscles, loss of muscle tone and tendon reflexes.

Following cord injury there is initially a state of *spinal shock*, characterized by flaccid paralysis below the lesion, loss of reflexes and retention of urine. As this subsides spastic paralysis ensues, with uninhibited flexor reflexes; slight stimulation of the foot provokes gross flexor spasms. An *automatic bladder* usually develops whereby, through sacral reflexes, it empties when distended. Lesions of the conus medullaris or cauda equina interrupt the central connexions of the bladder which then becomes *atonic*, distension causing incontinence.

Chapter 5

Brainstem

TRANSITION FROM SPINAL CORD TO MEDULLA OBLONGATA

In study of the brainstem it is helpful to consider initially how the grey and white matter of the cervical spinal cord are rearranged in the medulla. This transition is illustrated in *Fig.* 5.1.

White Matter

In the medulla, *corticospinal fibres* are located ventrally and bilaterally in the pyramids. As they descend through the *pyramidal decussation*, fibres forming a *lateral corticospinal tract* incline dorsolaterally into the lateral funiculus, and thus cut through the grey matter, isolating the ventral horn.

The nuclei gracilis and cuneatus, on the dorsal medullary aspect, mark the rostral extent of the spinal dorsal columns. Their axons arch ventromedially as *internal arcuate fibres* of the *sensory decussation*, which cross to form the opposite *medial lemniscus*, dorsal to the pyramid. This decussation also intersects grey matter, separating the medullary equivalent of the dorsal horn from central grey matter.

Two tracts in the spinal ventral funiculus are displaced dorsally in the medulla by the pyramid and medial lemniscus; these are the *tectospinal tract* and the *medial vestibulospinal tract* (medial longitudinal fasciculus in brainstem).

As the tracts are traced upwards in a lateral funiculus, a *dorsal spinocerebellar tract* enters the inferior cerebellar peduncle, and a *ventral spinocerebellar tract* passes through the medulla and pons to enter the superior peduncle. The remaining tracts (excluding corticospinal fibres, already described) are grouped dorsal to the inferior olivary nucleus. The *lateral and ventral spinothalamic and spinotectal tracts* are close, and are sometimes collectively termed the 'spinal lemniscus'. Extrapyramidal tracts – *rubrospinal, lateral vestibulospinal and reticulospinal* – are also located here, together with the *visceral efferent* pathway.

Grey matter

Although the spinal pattern of grey matter is altered in the medulla, there are functional similarities.

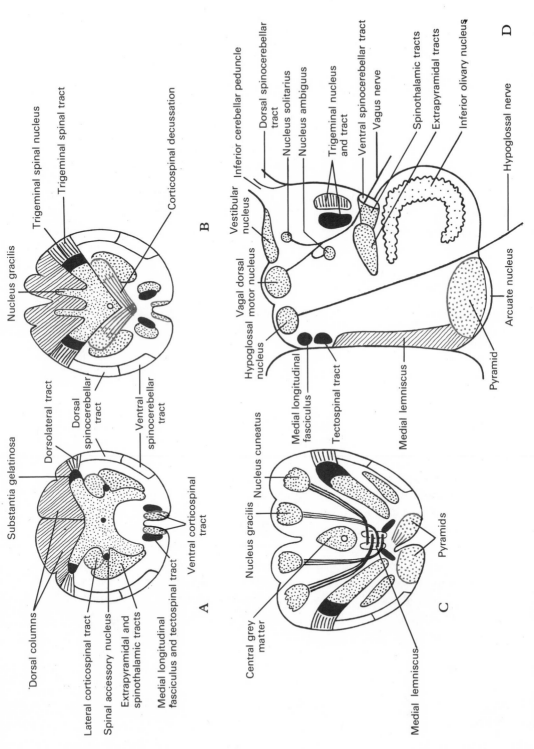

Fig. 5.1 Transition from spinal cord to medulla oblongata. (A) Segment C1 of spinal cord. (B) Medulla, level of corticospinal decussation. (C) Medulla, level of sensory decussation. (D) Medulla, level of olive.

Motor nerve roots emerge from the upper cervical cord in two separate rows for muscles of dissimilar developmental origin. The ventral nerve roots supply myotomal muscles: the *hypoglossal (XII)* nerve rootlets are in series with these and are equivalent to them. Other fibres emerge more dorsally from the lateral spinal aspect to form the *spinal accessory (XI)* nerve, ascending through the foramen magnum to supply the branchial arch musculature. The *cranial roots of the accessory (XI), vagus (X)* and *glossopharyngeal (IX)* nerves also supply branchial muscles: their roots emerge from the medulla in series with the spinal accessory nerve and are therefore posterior to the hypoglossal roots.

In the first two cervical spinal segments the nucleus proprius, substantia gelatinosa and tract of Lissauer blend with, and are largely replaced by, the *spinal nucleus and tract of the trigeminal (V) nerve.* The trigeminal tract, external to the nucleus, contains descending fibres from the facial region, concerned with pain and temperature sensation. The thoracic nucleus (nucleus dorsalis) has its medullary equivalent in the *accessory cuneate nucleus.*

Visceral afferent and efferent components of cranial nerves are parasympathetic, and are represented in the vagal and glossopharyngeal medullary nuclei. The vagus provides a widespread parasympathetic distribution in the thorax and abdomen. In contrast to the spinal cord, there is no sympathetic outflow in the cranial nerves. Sympathetic supply to the head and neck ascends from upper thoracic nerves to relay in cervical ganglia.

GENERAL TOPOGRAPHY OF THE BRAINSTEM

The brainstem is divisible for description into medulla, pons and midbrain (*Figs. 5.2, 5.3*).

The medulla

This is slightly conical, wider rostrally, extending from the lower pontine border to continue as the spinal cord immediately below the foramen magnum. The spinal central canal continues into the lower half of the medulla and then into the *fourth ventricle.* From the dorsal aspect the medulla has a *lower closed part,* and an *upper open part* in the floor of the fourth ventricle.

The spinal *ventral median fissure* continues to the pontine lower border, but in the lower medulla it is interrupted by the *decussation of the pyramids.* The spinal *dorsal median sulcus* extends into the lower medulla, separating the fasciculi graciles. Fibres of the hypoglossal nerve emerge from a *ventrolateral sulcus.* The cranial accessory, vagus and glossopharyngeal nerves have a row of rootlets at the *dorsolateral sulcus.* The medulla may be subdivided by these sulci into bilateral ventral, lateral and dorsal regions.

Ventrally, on each side of the median fissure, is the longitudinal elevation of a *pyramid,* composed of corticospinal fibres, most crossing in the pyramidal decussation to form a lateral corticospinal tract in the lateral funiculus, the rest continuing into the

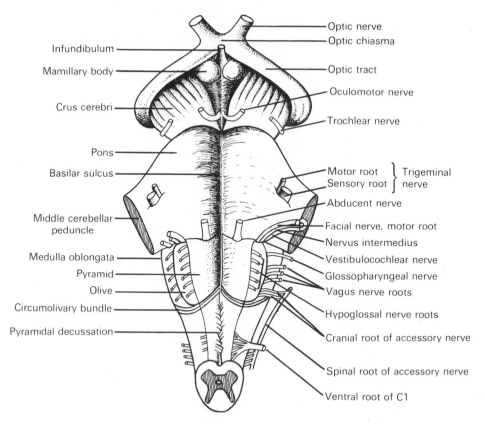

Fig. 5.2 Ventral aspect of the brainstem showing cranial nerves.

ventral funiculus as the ventral corticospinal tract. The *abducent (VI)* nerve emerges between the pyramid and pons.

Lateral to each pyramid, and separated from it by rootlets of the *hypoglossal (XII)* nerve, is the *olive*, an oval bulge made by a crumpled mass of grey matter, the *inferior olivary nucleus*. Nerve fibres emerge from the ventral median fissure, curving round the olive as the *circumolivary bundle* en route to the inferior cerebellar peduncle; these arise in the *arcuate nucleus*, superficial to the pyramid. Lateral to the olive, rootlets of the *glossopharyngeal (IX), vagus (X) and cranial accessory (XI) nerves* emerge, the last being joined by the spinal accessory nerve. In the angle between the lateral medulla and lower pontine border, the *facial (VII)* and *vestibulocochlear (VIII)* nerves appear: the facial is the more medial of the two and between them is the *nervus intermedius*, the so-called 'sensory root' of the facial nerve.

The dorsal surface of the lower half of medulla bilaterally comprises the terminations of fasciculi gracilis and cuneatus, which end in two ovoid *gracile and cuneate tubercles*, produced by the corresponding nuclei. Between the olive and lower part of the fourth ventricle on each side, an *inferior cerebellar peduncle* appears and bends dorsally as it ascends, forming the lower lateral boundary of the ventricle: it here receives the *striae medullares*, fibres originating in the arcuate nucleus and penetrating the medulla in the

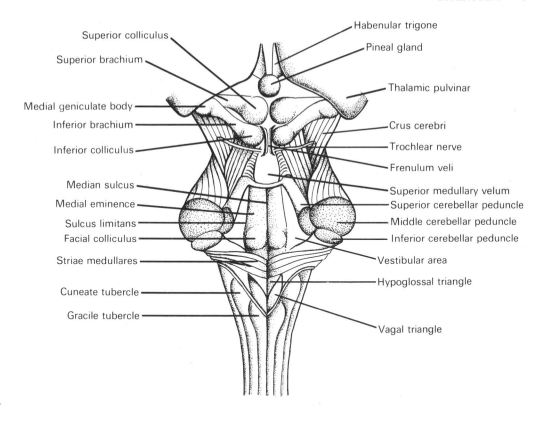

Fig. 5.3 Dorsal aspect of the brainstem and the floor of the fourth ventricle.

midline as they pass dorsally to cross the ventricular floor en route to the cerebellum. Efferent fibres from the arcuate nucleus are hence visible on the medullary surface both ventrally (circumolivary bundle) and dorsally (striae medullares).

The pons

The pons is between the medulla and the midbrain. Its prominent, convex, ventral, basilar surface is marked by transverse fibres, converging from numerous *pontine nuclei* to form a *middle cerebellar peduncle* on each side. The pontopeduncular transition is arbitrarily set at the attachment of the *trigeminal (V) nerve*. This nerve has two components; a small motor root is anteromedial to a larger sensory root. A shallow midline ventral *basilar sulcus* adjoins the basilar artery. The dorsal pontine surface forms the rostral half of the fourth ventricle's floor. When the internal pontine structure is described it will be evident that its dorsal region, *tegmentum* and ventral *basilar part* are quite different in content. The tegmentum is continuous rostrally with that of the midbrain, and caudally with the medulla, conveying tracts between them and containing some cranial nerve nuclei. Pyramidal tracts descend through the basilar region, broken into bundles by transverse pontocerebellar fibres.

The fourth ventricle

During hindbrain development, combined ventral flexure and dorsal cerebellar growth cause the neural tube to widen and flatten. The alar laminae of its lateral walls are splayed apart, like opening a book, and the roof plate is greatly attenuated (*Fig.* 5.4). Grey matter forms its floor; on each side the basal (motor) lamina is medial, the alar (sensory) lamina lateral and the sulcus limitans between them. Thus, in the floor of the fourth ventricle, somatic motor nuclei of the cranial nerves are near the midline, somatic sensory nuclei are lateral, and visceral components are intermediate around the sulcus limitans.

The *rhomboid fossa*, or fourth ventricular floor, is formed by the posterior surfaces of the pons and the open part of the medulla. Between the midbrain aqueduct rostrally and central canal of the medulla caudally, its lateral boundaries are formed by the superior cerebellar peduncles, inferior peduncles and cuneate and gracile tubercles (*Fig.* 5.3). At its widest level it has a *lateral recess* on each side. The floor is divided longitudinally by a *median sulcus*, from which *striae medullares* cross into lateral recesses, their position dividing the floor into pontine and medullary regions. Rostral to them, between the median sulcus and the sulcus limitans, is a ridge, the *medial eminence*, in whose lower part a slight swelling, the *facial colliculus*, is produced by facial nerve motor fibres looping over the abducent nucleus. The sensory region lateral to the sulcus limitans overlies the vestibular nuclear complex, and is hence the *vestibular area*. Caudal to the striae are two motor nuclei: adjacent to the midline is an eminence, the *hypoglossal triangle*; lateral to this the *vagal triangle* is a shallow depression like an inverted 'V'. These features, likened to a pen-nib, are collectively termed the 'calamus scriptorius'. These triangles mark the rostral end of the hypoglossal and vagal motor nuclei.

The roof of the fourth ventricle is angled in sagittal section (*Fig.* 5.5) and closely related to the cerebellum. Rostrally the *superior medullary velum* extends between the two superior cerebellar peduncles and meets the midbrain tectum. The cerebellum's lingula is fused with its dorsal surface. The caudal part of the roof is a very thin lamina of fused pia and ependyma, attached laterally to the posterior medullary surface to form the inferior boundary of the lateral recess. The caudal roof is deficient centrally as the

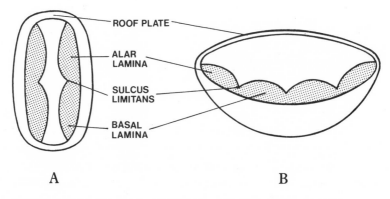

A   B

Fig. 5.4 Diagrammatic transverse sections comparing the developing neural tube in the spinal cord (A) and in the region of the fourth ventricle (B).

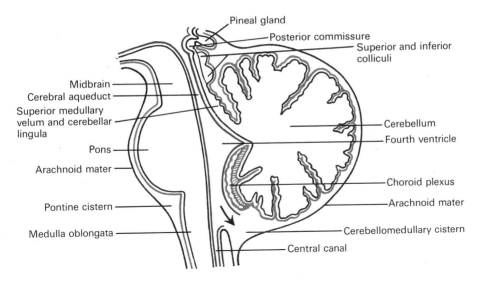

Fig. 5.5 Diagram of a sagittal section through the brainstem and cerebellum. The arrow is in the median aperture of the fourth ventricle. Ependyma in blue, pia mater in red.

median aperture of the fourth ventricle (foramen of Magendie) through which cerebrospinal fluid, formed in the ventricular system, escapes into the subarachnoid space. The lateral recesses lead to two smaller *lateral openings* (foramina of Luschka). The pia mater of the vascularized inferior velum forms a double fold, the *tela choroidea*, containing *choroid plexuses* of the fourth ventricle. These invaginate the roof, and its ependyma becomes secretory epithelium. The plexuses form the shape of a letter T, its vertical limb double as a convoluted vascular projection flanking the midline and extending caudally almost to the median aperture. The horizontal part extends into each lateral recess, commonly protruding through the lateral apertures.

The midbrain

The mesencephalon, about 2 cm in length and the shortest brainstem segment, connects the pons and cerebellum to the cerebrum and traverses the tentorial hiatus. For description it is divided sagittally into two *cerebral peduncles*, each consisting of an anterior *crus cerebri* (basis pedunculi) and posterior *tegmentum*. Between these is a stratum of pigmented cells, the *substantia nigra*.

The two crura cerebri, diverging anteriorly from the midline, consist of fibres descending from the ipsilateral cerebral cortex, namely the corticospinal, corticobulbar and corticopontine fibres. Between the crura is the *interpeduncular fossa*, the floor of which is known as the *posterior perforated substance*, penetrated by small arteries: the two *oculomotor (III) nerves* emerge from the fossa's sides. A *lateral sulcus* grooves each peduncle.

The *cerebral aqueduct* traverses the tegmentum, connecting the third and fourth ventricles. The region dorsal to the plane of the aqueduct is the *tectum*, or roof, occupied externally by four paired, round elevations, the *superior and inferior colliculi* (corpora quadrigemina). From the caudal end of the tectum a white median fold, the *frenulum veli*, extends to the superior medullary velum, on each side of which a fine *trochlear (IV) nerve* emerges and curves ventrally round the midbrain. The inferior colliculi are relay stations on auditory pathways. From each inferior colliculus, ascending fibres form an elevated *inferior brachium* as they pass to a thalamic nucleus, the *medial geniculate body*. The superior colliculi are concerned with visual reflexes; a *superior brachium* extends to each from a *lateral geniculate body*, containing descending fibres from the optic tract and visual cortex (retinocollicular and corticocollicular).

INTERNAL STRUCTURE OF THE BRAINSTEM

The locations of the cranial nerve nuclei will be detailed later; we are here concerned with the general internal plan, best studied in representative sections to construct a three-dimensional concept. For convenience, each photograph has been bisected and half is shown diagrammatically (*Figs.* 5.6–5.14).

The medulla

In the lowest medullary levels (*Fig.* 5.6) the ventral grey column is separated from the central grey matter by decussating corticospinal fibres; as these descend, most pass dorsolaterally in the pyramidal decussation. The 'detached' ventral grey column contains the *nucleus ambiguus*, the branchiomotor component of the cranial accessory nerve at this level, and of the vagus and glossopharyngeal nerves more rostrally; it supplies striated muscle. The *dorsal motor vagal nucleus* (parasympathetic), which supplies smooth muscle, is located in the central grey matter. The general visceral afferent components of both vagus nerves meet dorsal to the central canal as the median *commissural nucleus*. Upward continuation of the dorsal grey horn is represented here by the *spinal trigeminal nucleus*, bounded peripherally by its afferent tract. The *nucleus gracilis* is beginning to appear in the corresponding funiculus.

A transverse section just above the pyramidal decussation (*Fig.* 5.7) shows a development of these features, and some new structures. The *sensory decussation* of the internal arcuate fibres streams ventromedially from the nucleus gracilis and nucleus cuneatus, crossing the midline to form the contralateral *medial lemniscus*; the somatotopic arrangement in it is such that input from the lower half of the body, via the fasciculus gracilis, is ventral to that from the nucleus cuneatus. The *trigeminal nucleus* is separated from the central grey matter by the sensory decussation. The *medial longitudinal fasciculus* lies dorsal to the medial lemniscus. The *accessory cuneate nucleus* (comparable to the thoracic nucleus) receives proprioceptive input from upper cervical segments, projecting to the cerebellum via the inferior peduncle. The central canal has inclined dorsally, prior to its junction with the fourth ventricle. The central grey matter contains medially the *hypoglossal nucleus*, lateral to which are vagal components including the *nucleus solitarius*. Flanked by its own afferent tract, the latter subserves

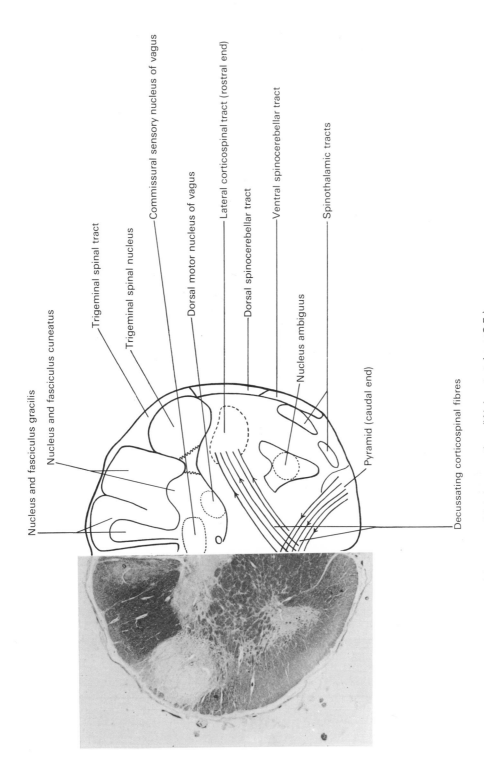

Fig. 5.6 Medulla at the level of the pyramidal decussation. (Weigert stain, ×8.5.)

Nucleus and fasciculus gracilis

Nucleus and fasciculus cuneatus

Trigeminal spinal tract

Trigeminal spinal nucleus

Commissural sensory nucleus of vagus

Dorsal motor nucleus of vagus

Lateral corticospinal tract (rostral end)

Dorsal spinocerebellar tract

Ventral spinocerebellar tract

Spinothalamic tracts

Nucleus ambiguus

Pyramid (caudal end)

Decussating corticospinal fibres

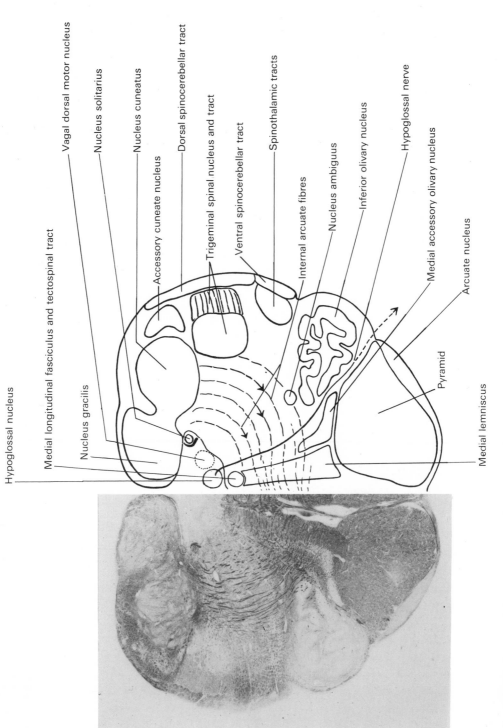

Fig. 5.7 Medulla at the level of the sensory decussation. (Weigert stain, ×6.5.)

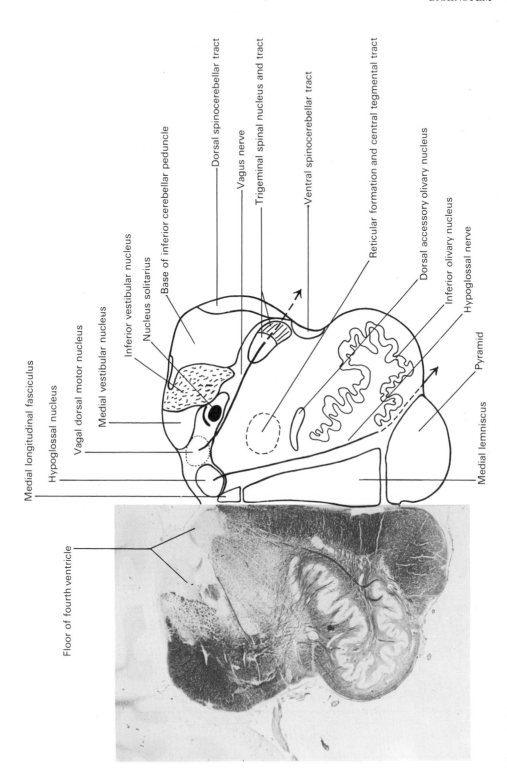

Medial longitudinal fasciculus

Hypoglossal nucleus

Vagal dorsal motor nucleus

Medial vestibular nucleus

Inferior vestibular nucleus

Nucleus solitarius

Base of inferior cerebellar peduncle

Dorsal spinocerebellar tract

Vagus nerve

Trigeminal spinal nucleus and tract

Ventral spinocerebellar tract

Reticular formation and central tegmental tract

Dorsal accessory olivary nucleus

Inferior olivary nucleus

Hypoglossal nerve

Pyramid

Medial lemniscus

Floor of fourth ventricle

Fig. 5.8 Medulla at mid-olivary level. (Weigert stain, ×5.5.)

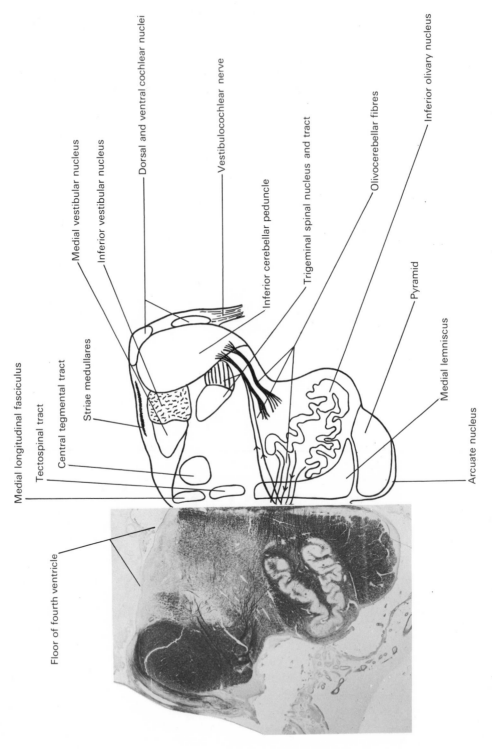

Fig. 5.9 Rostral end of the medulla. (Weigert stain, ×4.5.)

taste sensation mediated by nerves VII, IX and X. There are additional areas of grey matter: the *arcuate nucleus* overlies the pyramid, representing 'displaced' pontine nuclei in the cortico-ponto-cerebellar pathway; the caudal extremity of *inferior olivary nucleus* is dorsolateral to the pyramid. Throughout the medulla is the *reticular formation*, a diffuse network of cells and fine fibres, to be described later.

In the next section (*Fig. 5.8*), the central grey matter has opened out into the fourth ventricle. The *hypoglossal nucleus* is flanked by the *dorsal vagal motor nucleus* and the *nucleus solitarius* and its tract. The medial and inferior *vestibular nuclei* are lateral in the ventricular floor. The *inferior cerebellar peduncle* has received the dorsal spinocerebellar tract, and overlies the trigeminal nucleus and tract. The *inferior olivary nucleus* is a large hollow grey mass with a medial open hilum from which *olivocerebellar fibres* pass to the opposite inferior cerebellar peduncle. The dorsal and medial *accessory olivary nuclei* are phylogenetically more ancient. The inferior olivary complex will be described later in relation to the cerebellum. The *hypoglossal nerve* passes lateral to the medial lemniscus to emerge between the pyramid and olive. The *vagus nerve* penetrates the trigeminal nucleus to emerge dorsal to the olive. The hypoglossal nerve demarcates the medulla into areas of different blood supply; the area medial to it is supplied by the anterior spinal artery, the area dorsolateral to it by the posterior inferior cerebellar artery. The *spinothalamic tracts*, *extrapyramidal tracts* (vestibulospinal, reticulospinal and rubrospinal), the *visceral efferent pathway* and the *nucleus ambiguus* are all in the area dorsal to the inferior olivary nucleus and, together with the vestibular nuclei, are damaged by thrombosis of the posterior inferior cerebellar artery.

A section at the cranial end of the medulla (*Fig. 5.9*) shows some features already noted. The ventricular floor has widened and *striae medullares* traverse it at the pontomedullary junction. The inferior cerebellar peduncle is larger and the *dorsal and ventral cochlear nuclei* adjoin it. The *vestibulocochlear nerve* emerges in the cerebello-medullary angle. The medial lemniscus is beginning to extend between the pyramid and inferior olive; at the pontomedullary junction it rotates through 90° into a transverse plane.

The pons

The next three sections (*Figs. 5.10, 5.11, 5.12*) are at levels through the facial nucleus, trigeminal nerve, and rostral pons. In each, the basilar region contains *descending fasciculi* (corticospinal, corticobulbar and corticopontine), interspersed with *transverse fibres* from numerous nuclei pontis forming the *middle cerebellar peduncles*. The fourth ventricle is flanked by the *superior cerebellar peduncles* and roofed by the superior medullary velum, overlain by the cerebellar lingula. Each superior peduncle is the efferent path from a large intracerebellar dentate nucleus, which projects to the opposite red nucleus in the midbrain, and thence to the thalamus. This dentato-rubro-thalamic path is the route by which the cerebellum influences cerebral cortical motor activity.

In the first section (*Fig. 5.10*), the inferior cerebellar peduncle has turned dorsally and is between the other peduncles. Deep to the ventricular floor, each side of the midline throughout the pons and medulla, is the *medial longitudinal fasciculus*, an

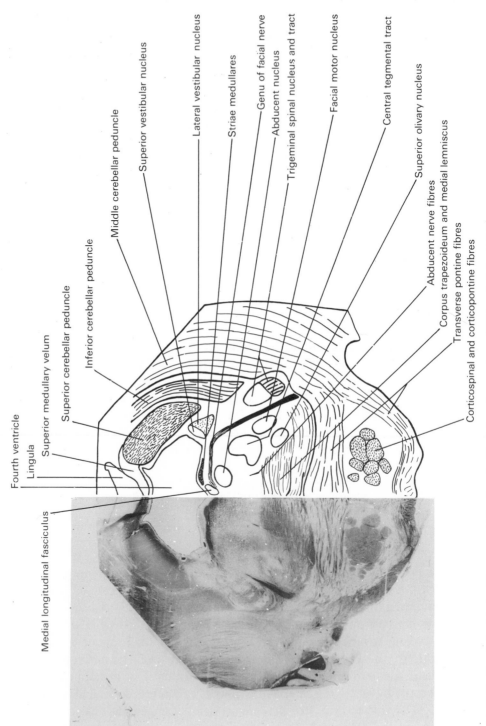

Fourth ventricle
Lingula
Superior medullary velum
Superior cerebellar peduncle
Inferior cerebellar peduncle
Middle cerebellar peduncle
Superior vestibular nucleus
Lateral vestibular nucleus
Striae medullares
Genu of facial nerve
Abducent nucleus
Trigeminal spinal nucleus and tract
Facial motor nucleus
Central tegmental tract
Superior olivary nucleus
Abducent nerve fibres
Corpus trapezoideum and medial lemniscus
Transverse pontine fibres
Corticospinal and corticopontine fibres
Medial longitudinal fasciculus

Fig. 5.10 Caudal region of the pons at the level of facial motor nucleus. (Weigert stain, × 2.8).

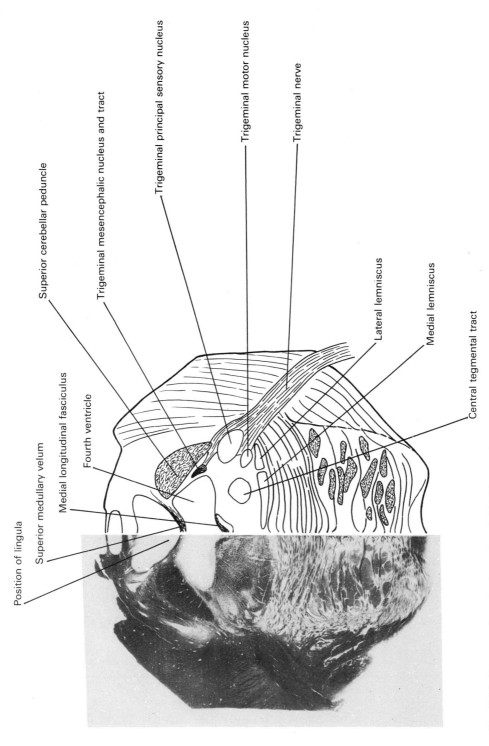

Fig. 5.11 Pons at trigeminal root level. (Weigert stain, × 2.5.)

Position of lingula

Superior medullary velum

Medial longitudinal fasciculus

Fourth ventricle

Superior cerebellar peduncle

Trigeminal mesencephalic nucleus and tract

Trigeminal principal sensory nucleus

Trigeminal motor nucleus

Trigeminal nerve

Lateral lemniscus

Medial lemniscus

Central tegmental tract

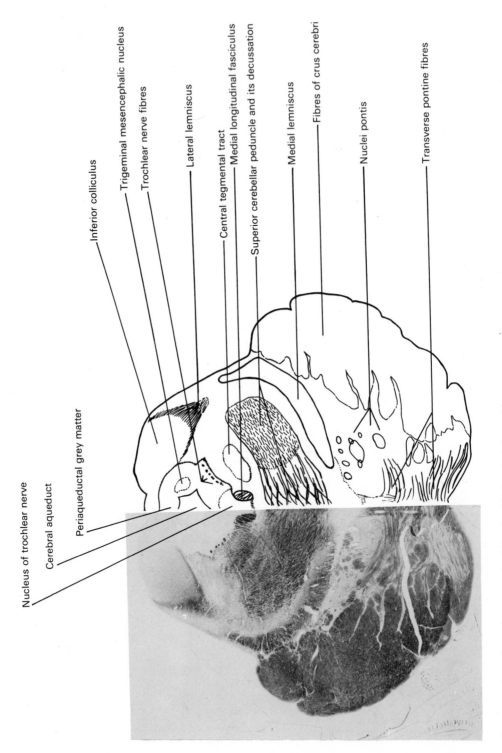

Fig. 5.12 Junction of pons and midbrain. (Weigert stain, × 4.)

association tract between the nuclei controlling eye muscles (oculogyric nuclei) and the vestibular nuclei. It ascends in the midbrain to the interstitial nucleus, and descends in the spinal cord to the spinal accessory nucleus, and thus is sometimes termed the 'interstitiospinal tract'; caudally it continues into the medial vestibulospinal tract, co-ordinating movements of the head, eyes and neck; it will be considered further with the eighth cranial nerve. The *facial colliculus* is formed by fibres from the *facial motor nucleus* curving over the abducent nucleus. The facial nerve's efferent path is between its motor nucleus and the *trigeminal sensory nucleus and tract*. The *vestibular nuclei* are near the lateral angle of the ventricular floor. The *medial lemniscus*, joined by trigemino-thalamic and spinothalamic fibres, lies horizontally, intersected by transverse auditory fibres, forming the *corpus trapezoideum*. The *superior olivary nucleus* is also associated with the auditory path.

Fig. 5.11 illustrates a section through the *trigeminal nerve*; its *motor nucleus* is medial to its *principal sensory nucleus*. The trigeminal *mesencephalic tract* carries proprioceptive fibres, ascending alongside the narrowed ventricular cavity en route to the midbrain. The *reticular formation* is present throughout the pontine tegmentum, and the *central tegmental tract* is a relatively dense group of fibres in it, ascending to the thalamus and descending to the inferior olivary nucleus. Two reticular nuclei have particular significance. The *locus caeruleus* lies ventral to the mesencephalic trigeminal nucleus. It is a source of noradrenaline (norepinephrine), and has remarkably widespread projections throughout the central nervous system. Its thalamic and cortical connexions play a role in 'paradoxical sleep'. The midline *raphé nuclei* produce serotonin (5–HT) which, in general, has an inhibitory effect. Descending fibres inhibit pain transmission; ascending fibres are associated with 'slow wave sleep'; destruction of the raphé nuclei produces insomnia. The cells of the locus caeruleus and raphé nuclei are readily distinguished by the formaldehyde-fluorescence technique: noradrenaline fluoresces pale green and serotonin yellow.

At the junction of the pons and midbrain (*Fig.* 5.12), where the fourth ventricle and aqueduct join, the *superior cerebellar peduncles* decussate. The *medial lemniscus* has moved away from the midline and the *lateral lemniscus* inclines dorsally to enter the inferior colliculus. In the basilar region descending fibres are massed together rather than scattered in bundles.

The midbrain

Each *crus cerebri* (basis pedunculi) is separated from the tegmentum by the *substantia nigra*, which extends from the lateral midbrain sulcus to the interpeduncular fossa. The substantia nigra is a large extrapyramidal nucleus: the black colour seen in unstained sections is due to melanin, a precursor in dopamine metabolism. Dopamine is deficient in Parkinson's disease, an extrapyramidal disorder which will be described in Chapter 9. Each crus cerebri consists of descending fibres, *corticospinal* and *corticobulbar* fibres occupying its middle two thirds, the latter including corticonuclear fibres to cranial nerve motor nuclei. Here the somatotopic arrangement is such that the head is medial and the feet lateral. *Corticopontine* fibres have extensive origins in the cerebral cortex and

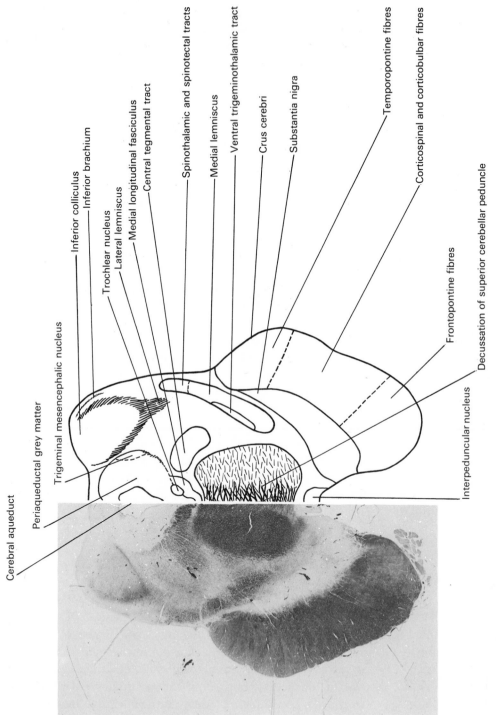

Fig. 5.13 Lower midbrain at the level of the inferior colliculus. (Weigert stain, ×5.)

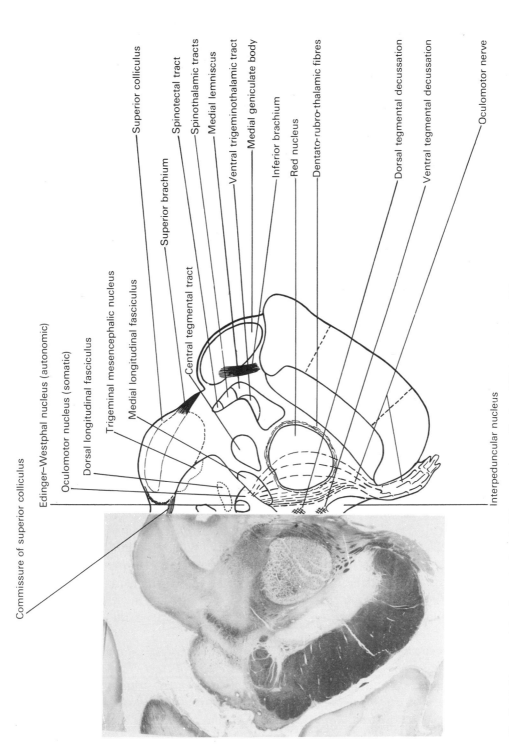

Fig. 5.14 Upper midbrain at the level of the superior colliculus. (Weigert stain, × 3.)

descend to synapse ipsilaterally with the nuclei pontis; in the crus cerebri they are in two main groups, lateral temporopontine and medial frontopontine.

A section at inferior collicular level (*Fig.* 5.13) shows features differing from those in sections through the superior colliculus (*Fig.* 5.14). In the more caudal section (*Fig.* 5.13) the *lateral lemniscus* is passing into the *inferior colliculus*, a relay point on the auditory path. The *medial lemniscus* inclines dorsally en route to the thalamus. The *decussation of the superior cerebellar peduncles* is a prominent central feature. The *trochlear nucleus* is ventral in the periaqueductal grey matter, contiguous with the *medial longitudinal fasciculus*; it supplies the ocular superior oblique muscle and its fibres pass dorsally, crossing the midline before emerging from the superior medullary velum. The *mesencephalic trigeminal tract*, being sensory, is more dorsal in the grey matter. The *mesencephalic nucleus* of the trigeminal nerve consists of unipolar cells which are primary sensory neurons, unique in this central location (cf. spinal dorsal root ganglion).

At the level of the *superior colliculus* (*Fig.* 5.14) is the *red nucleus*, a large round mass on each side, continuous with the crossed superior cerebellar peduncle. It has a pinkish colour in fresh sections. Some fibres of the dentato-rubro-thalamic tract terminate in it, while others surround it in their onward path to the thalamus. The red nucleus is extrapyramidal, its fibres crossing in the *ventral tegmental decussation* to form the rubrospinal tract; the nucleus also provides a large input to the reticular formation. The *superior colliculi* have a complex, seven-layered structure of grey and white matter, reflecting their derivation from the optic lobes of lower vertebrates. In man they are concerned in visual reflexes and eye movements, integrating afferents from diverse sources – cortical, retinal (via the superior brachium), auditory (from the inferior colliculus) and spinal. Descending fibres, originating in the superior colliculus, cross in the *dorsal tegmental decussation* to form the tectospinal and tectobulbar tracts. Tectobulbar connexions influence the oculogyric nuclei (controlling reflex eye movements) and the facial motor nuclei (controlling reflex closure of the eyelids). Interconnexions between the superior colliculi form part of the *posterior commissure*. The pretectal nucleus, not seen in this section, is anterolateral to the superior colliculus, participating in the pupillary reflex response to light. These structures will be described with the oculogyric nuclei (III, IV, VI). The *inferior brachium*, ascending from the inferior colliculus to the medial geniculate body, forms a dorsolateral ridge on the midbrain surface. The *oculomotor nucleus* is ventral in the periaqueductal grey matter, near the *medial longitudinal fasciculus*; it supplies four extra-ocular muscles and striated muscle of the levator palpebrae superioris. Its dorsal region contains a parasympathetic component, the *Edinger-Westphal nucleus*, innervating the ciliary muscle and constrictor pupillae. Oculomotor fibres traverse the red nucleus to emerge in the interpeduncular fossa.

Autonomic pathways descend from the hypothalamus through the midbrain. From the hypothalamic mamillary bodies, the *mamillotegmental tract* enters the tegmental reticular formation and thence, via polysynaptic fibres, extends through the brainstem to spinal cord. The *dorsal longitudinal fasciculus* consists of non-myelinated fibres in the periaqueductal grey matter, descending to autonomic nuclei of the brainstem. The *interpeduncular nucleus* of the midbrain is in an efferent path from the habenular nucleus (situated rostral to the superior colliculus); it is associated with olfaction and, through various cranial nerve nuclei, it influences salivation, gastric secretion and gastrointestinal motility.

THE RETICULAR FORMATION

The primitive vertebrate brain is a diffuse network of nerve cells and fibres; it persists in the human central nervous system between subsequently developed nuclei and tracts. It is polyneuronal and polysynaptic. In the brainstem its very long fibres are transverse, each bifurcating into a long ascending and long descending branch, with many collaterals, allowing widespread interactions. It is non-specific as regards modalities, but serves somatic and visceral functions. Its ascending and descending fibres are crossed and uncrossed; experimental analysis of these is difficult, since their polysynaptic nature does not favour degeneration techniques.

In the brainstem, groups of nerve cells in the reticular formation are referred to as nuclei, which have been classified in various ways. Their descending spinal paths may inhibit or facilitate ventral horn cells. In the medulla there are lateral and medial groups; the *lateral reticular nucleus* is dorsolateral to the inferior olivary nucleus, the *medial reticular nucleus* lies near the central tegmental tract, and in the midline there are scattered elements constituting the *nucleus of the raphé*. Experimental stimulation of the latter inhibits pain perception, probably by an effect on input mediated by fibres descending to the spinal dorsal grey column. These reticular nuclei extend rostrally into the pons and midbrain; in the latter there are also periaqueductal reticular nuclei. The *locus caeruleus* and upper raphé nuclei have already been described.

Input to the brainstem reticular formation from all forms of sensation, somatic and visceral, is diffuse; it includes ascending spinal tracts (except the dorsal column-medial lemniscal path which is discrete and discriminatory) and sensory components of cranial nerve nuclei, particularly the trigeminal, vestibular and cochlear. The cerebellum and the medullary reticular formation are closely associated via the inferior peduncles. Descending connexions from the cerebral cortex are via corticoreticular fibres and collaterals from corticospinal and corticobulbar tracts. The hypothalamus, limbic system and some extrapyramidal nuclei such as the red nucleus also produce effects via the reticular formation.

The ascending *reticular activating system* projects through thalamic nuclei to the cerebral cortex and is involved in arousal, alerting reactions and heightened perception. Pain, loud noises or strong psychic stimuli thus inhibit sleep. Prolonged coma may follow damage to this system. Anaesthesia or barbiturates block transmission through the polysynaptic reticular paths and the cortex thus becomes unresponsive to impulses which still arrive via specific sensory pathways. Natural sleep should not, however, be regarded as simply passive; there are *hypnogenic zones* in the brainstem reticular formation.

Descending *reticulospinal tracts* especially influence activity in γ reflex loops and also end near α motor neurons. The medial part of the medullary reticular formation is inhibitory; the larger lateral region, extending through the pons to midbrain, is excitatory.

Respiratory and *cardiovascular* functions are influenced by the so-called 'vital centres' in the medullary and lower pontine reticular formation. Higher control is mediated through these centres from the hypothalamus. Trauma to the brainstem is often lethal due to damage in these centres.

APPLIED ANATOMY

Vascular lesions of the brainstem illustrate the location of nuclei and tracts. The main blood suppliers are the two vertebral arteries, joining at the pontomedullary junction to form the basilar artery, which extends rostrally to divide into two posterior cerebral arteries. The vertebral arteries each supply a medial branch to form the anterior spinal artery: this supplies the medial part of the medulla and the cervical spinal cord. From the lateral aspect of each vertebral artery, a posterior inferior cerebellar artery winds round the side of the medulla to supply the dorsolateral region.

The *medial medullary syndrome* is a result of blockage of the anterior spinal artery or medial medullary branches of the vertebral artery. It affects the pyramid, medial lemniscus and hypoglossal nerve (*Fig.* 5.15), resulting in contralateral hemiparesis of the limbs, ipsilateral lingual paralysis, and contralateral impaired perception of joint position, vibration and discriminative touch.

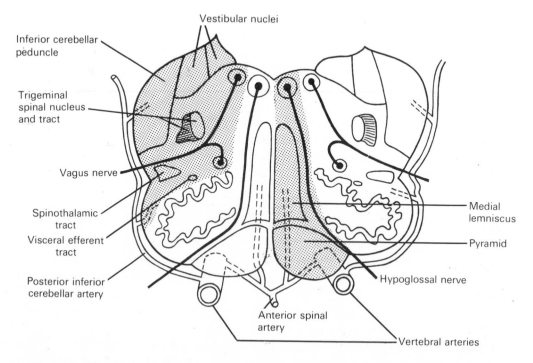

Fig. 5.15 Medullary infarction: (on left) of the posterior inferior cerebellar artery (lateral medullary syndrome); (on right) of the anterior spinal artery (medial medullary syndrome).

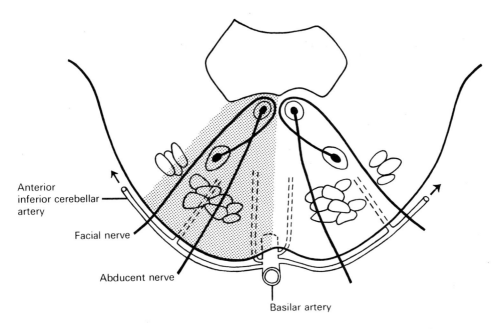

Fig. 5.16 Paramedian pontine infarction.

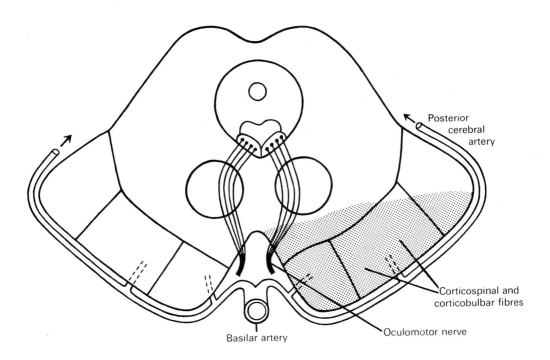

Fig. 5.17 Basal midbrain infarction.

The *lateral medullary syndrome* (*Fig.* 5.15) results from thrombosis of a posterior inferior cerebellar artery or a vertebral artery. This leads to severe dizziness (infarction of the vestibular nuclei), difficulty in swallowing and speaking (nucleus ambiguus), ipsilateral facial loss of pain and temperature sensation (trigeminal spinal nucleus), contralateral loss of pain and temperature sensation in the body (lateral spinothalamic tract), and Horner's syndrome (visceral efferent pathway). Ipsilateral ataxia follows impairment of blood supply to the inferior cerebellar peduncle and cerebellum.

Basal infarction of the pons (*Fig.* 5.16) follows occlusion of pontine branches of the basilar artery. Corticospinal fibres are dispersed at this level and partial contralateral hemiplegia results. Abducent nerve damage paralyses the lateral rectus muscle. If the lesion extends dorsally the facial nerve may be affected.

Basal midbrain lesion (*Fig.* 5.17) results from thrombosis of central branches of the posterior cerebral artery, involving corticospinal and corticobulbar fibres in the basis pedunculi, with contralateral hemiplegia. Destruction of the oculomotor nerve causes severe ipsilateral ophthalmoplegia, only the lateral rectus and superior oblique muscles escaping.

Internuclear ophthalmoplegia arises when the medial longitudinal fasciculus is involved either in a vascular lesion or in a demyelinating disease such as multiple sclerosis.

Chapter 6

Cranial nerves

The cranial nerves are numbered in rostrocaudal order:

I	–	Olfactory	VII	–	Facial
II	–	Optic	VIII	–	Vestibulocochlear
III	–	Oculomotor	IX	–	Glossopharyngeal
IV	–	Trochlear	X	–	Vagus
V	–	Trigeminal	XI	–	Accessory
VI	–	Abducent	XII	–	Hypoglossal

They may be classified into three main morphological groups:

1. Those supplying muscles derived from the cranial myotomes, namely the oculomotor (III), trochlear (IV) and abducent (VI) which supply the eye muscles, and the hypoglossal (XII) supplying the tongue.
2. Those innervating muscles of branchial origin, namely the trigeminal (V), facial (VII), glossopharyngeal (IX), vagus (X) and accessory (XI).
3. Those associated with special sense organs, namely the olfactory (I), optic (II) and vestibulocochlear (VIII). The olfactory and optic nerves are described separately in Chapters 10 and 11.

COMPONENTS

In the spinal nerves four 'general' components are found, namely the somatic and visceral afferent and the visceral and somatic efferent (*Fig.* 6.1A). These are represented singly or in combination in some cranial nerves, the visceral elements being parasympathetic only. In addition, three 'special' components are found in some cranial nerves (*Fig.* 6.1B). The vestibulocochlear fibres are *special somatic afferent*, associated with equilibration and hearing. Gustation (taste) is served by *special visceral afferent* fibres and nuclei of the facial, glossopharyngeal and vagus nerves. Branchiomotor nerves are regarded as *special visceral efferent*, since muscles of branchial origin in the face, mouth, pharynx and larynx are associated with visceral functions such as eating and breathing. There are therefore seven possible components in cranial nerves, though none contains all of these. Proprioceptive afferents in the cranial nerves probably all

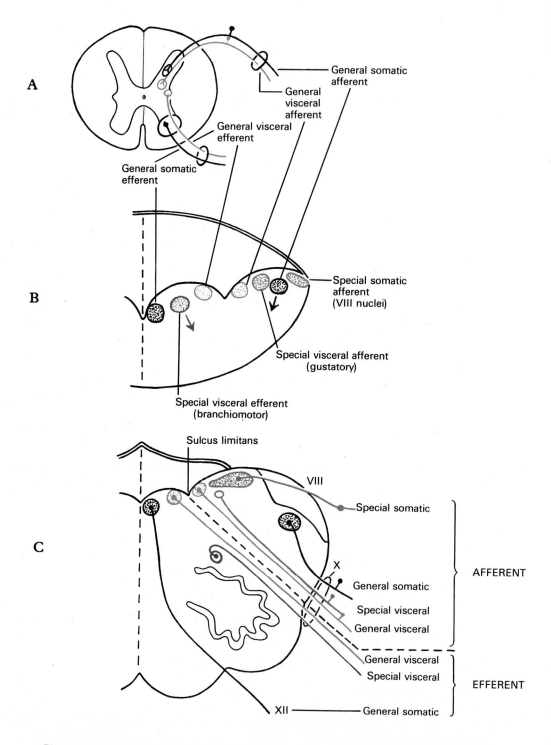

A

B

C

Fig. 6.1 Components of nerves. Compare spinal cord (A) with developing brainstem (B). (C) illustrates components of cranial nerves and their nuclei in the medulla. Black: general somatic. Green: general visceral. Red: special afferent. Blue: special efferent.

converge on a mesencephalic nucleus usually labelled as part of the trigeminal sensory complex.

As already noted in development of the fourth ventricle, grey matter forms its floor, white matter being ventral to this (*Fig.* 5.4). On each side the grey matter is divided by the sulcus limitans into a lateral sensory and a medial motor area. The disposition of the seven functional components of the cranial nerves is shown during development in *Fig.* 6.1B and their final locations in *Fig.* 6.1C. A large vestibular nuclear complex occupies much of the lateral part of the ventricular floor; the trigeminal sensory nucleus is displaced deeper in the medulla and pons. Most of the branchiomotor column migrates ventrolaterally during development, and the nucleus ambiguus ends just dorsal to the medial part of the inferior olive. The distributions of the sensory and motor nuclei are shown in *Figs.* 6.2 and 6.3: these are described with their cranial nerves.

General comparison of cranial and spinal nerves

It is useful to summarize certain generalizations at this stage:

1. Cranial nerves may contain 'special' components absent from spinal nerves.
2. Each (thoracic) spinal nerve contains four general components, but cranial nerves vary in both the number and the functional type of their components.
3. In the spinal cord there are four continuous columns of nuclei in the grey matter. In the brainstem the motor 'column' is in separated nuclei (*Fig.* 6.2). The trigeminal sensory nucleus, however, is a column from the midbrain to the cervical spinal cord (*Fig.* 6.3).
4. *Afferent ganglia.* The spinal dorsal root ganglia contain the cell bodies of visceral *and* somatic afferent neurons. If a cranial nerve has afferent fibres, the cell bodies of primary sensory neurons are also in ganglia, but these are usually either somatic *or* visceral. Thus the trigeminal ganglion is purely somatic afferent. The vagus and glossopharyngeal nerves each have two ganglia, a superior (mostly somatic) and an inferior (mostly visceral). The facial geniculate ganglion consists mostly of cell bodies of special visceral afferent neurons subserving taste, but a few of its cells mediate general somatic afferent sensation. The proprioceptive trigeminal input is unique: the cell bodies of the primary sensory neurons are in the midbrain (mesencephalic nucleus).
5. *Efferent ganglia.* Efferent parasympathetic components of cranial nerves synapse in peripheral ganglia (*Fig.* 6.2). Thus, for example, such efferent fibres in the oculomotor nerve synapse in the ciliary ganglion to supply the constrictor pupillae and ciliaris oculi. Vagal parasympathetic ganglia are scattered in plexuses in the walls of viscera.

The following descriptions of cranial nerves deal with their nuclear origins, central connexions, general course and distribution, function and dysfunction. They will be described in an ascending regional order in conformity with the sequence adopted in the account of the brainstem in Chapter 5.

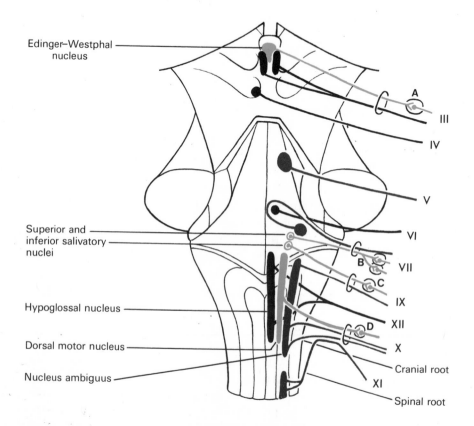

Fig. 6.2 Motor nuclei of the cranial nerves. Black: general somatic. Green: general visceral (parasympathetic). Blue: special visceral (branchiomotor). Parasympathetic ganglia: **A**, ciliary; **B**, pterygopalatine and submandibular; **C**, otic; **D**, peripheral visceral ganglia in thorax and abdomen.

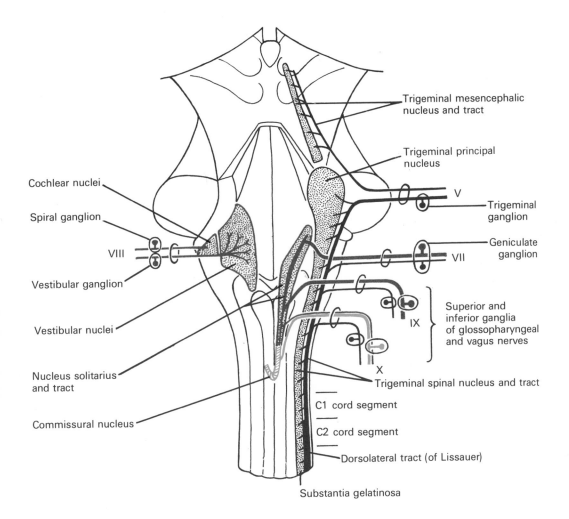

Fig. 6.3 Sensory nuclei and ganglia of the cranial nerves. Black: somatic. Green: general visceral. Red: special somatic, special visceral.

THE HYPOGLOSSAL (XII) NERVE

The *hypoglossal* nucleus is somatic efferent, in series with spinal ventral grey column cells. It is a column in the medulla, near the midline. Rostrally it underlies the hypoglossal triangle in the floor of the fourth ventricle and extends caudally into the ventral grey matter of the closed part of the medulla (*Fig.* 6.4). Fibres pass ventrally from the nucleus, lateral to the medial lemniscus, emerging as a row of 10–15 rootlets in the sulcus between the pyramid and the olive. The rootlets form two bundles, piercing the dura mater separately to traverse the hypoglossal canal in the occipital bone; since this is posteromedial to the jugular foramen, the emerging nerve is behind the internal jugular vein and associated cranial nerves (IX, X, XI). It descends laterally behind the vagus and glossopharyngeal nerves, passing forwards between the internal jugular vein and internal carotid artery and finally superficial to the internal and external carotid arteries to reach the lingual muscles (*Fig.* 6.4). It supplies the lingual intrinsic muscles and the extrinsic styloglossus, hyoglossus and genioglossus. It is joined by a communication from the anterior primary ramus of C1, the fibres of which the hypoglossal distributes to the geniohyoid and thyrohyoid; descending C1 fibres constitute the upper root of the *ansa cervicalis*, C2 and C3 fibres constituting its lower root.

Hypoglossal *central connexions* exemplify those typical of somatomotor nuclei of cranial nerves:
1. *Corticonuclear innervation.* This is mostly crossed; control of the genioglossus is entirely contralateral.
2. *Extrapyramidal afferents.*
3. *Associated sensory nuclei:* Reflex links with sensory input are comparable to spinal reflex arc connexions. For example, tongue movements may be responses to gustatory stimuli (via the nucleus solitarius) or to tactile oral stimuli (via the trigeminal sensory nuclei).
4. *Associated motor nuclei:* Movements of the facial, masticatory and pharyngeal muscles are co-ordinated by connexions between the motor nuclei of cranial nerves V, VII, IX, X, XI (cranial root), and XII.

APPLIED ANATOMY

As in lesions of spinal nerves, the results of lower motor neuron lesions (nuclear or infranuclear) differ from effects of upper motor neuron (supranuclear) lesions.

The degree of bilateral *supranuclear* innervation varies between individuals: an upper motor neuron lesion may cause contralateral or bilateral weakness; atrophy is slight or absent. Since the cortical innervation of the genioglossus is wholly contralateral, the tongue when protruded deviates away from the side of a unilateral lesion. Supranuclear damage in the internal capsule is usually vascular; corticonuclear fibres may degenerate in cerebral atherosclerosis. Tremor of the tongue is sometimes a feature in extra-pyramidal disease.

When the hypoglossal *nerve* is interrupted, half of the tongue atrophies; if protruded it deviates to the side of the lesion because of the unopposed action of the opposite genioglossus. The hypoglossal *nucleus* may be affected by vascular occlusion (*Fig.* 5.15), or in poliomyelitis.

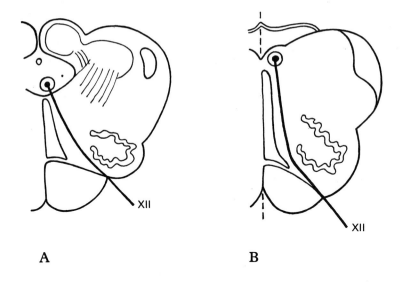

A

B

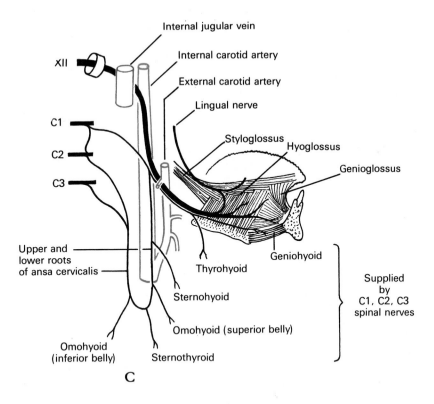

C

Fig. 6.4 The hypoglossal nerve. (A) Lower medulla. (B) Upper medulla. (C) Course and relationships.

THE ACCESSORY (XI) NERVE

The *accessory nerve* (*Fig.* 6.5) is branchiomotor and has *spinal* and *cranial* roots, which have separate origins and destinations, and are joined together for a short distance only in the jugular foramen. Beyond this the *cranial* root fuses with the vagus and is distributed by its pharyngeal and laryngeal branches to the soft palate, pharynx and larynx. It arises in the caudal part of the *nucleus ambiguus*, its rootlets emerging in line with those of the vagus, of which it is a part. The vagus and cranial accessory nerves will be described together.

The *spinal accessory nerve* starts from the *accessory nucleus*, a column of nerve cells dorsolateral in the ventral horn of the first five cervical segments. Morphologically, the rostral end of the accessory nucleus is probably in series with the nucleus ambiguus: whether the sternomastoid and trapezius muscles are of branchial arch origin is debatable. The nerve roots traverse the lateral funiculus, emerge between the dorsal and ventral spinal roots, and ascend posterior to the ligamenta denticulata. The nerve enters the posterior cranial fossa via the foramen magnum behind the vertebral artery, leaving through the jugular foramen, where it briefly adheres to its cranial root. It then descends laterally to the deep surface of the sternomastoid, emerges from the middle of the posterior border of the latter and crosses the posterior triangle to enter the trapezius

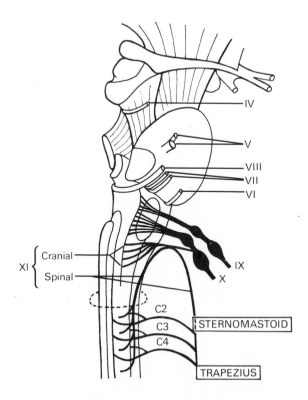

Fig. 6.5 Lateral view of the brainstem and upper cervical spinal cord. Note the cranial and spinal roots of the accessory nerve and the relationships of the former to the vagus. Cervical fibres to the trapezius are mostly sensory.

about 5 cm above the clavicle. The nerve is enclosed in the fascia of the triangle's roof, and is hence close to the superficial cervical lymph nodes. The third and fourth cervical spinal nerves supply the trapezius with proprioceptive fibres, and probably some motor fibres to its lower part.

APPLIED ANATOMY

The spinal accessory nerve's supranuclear control is unusual: it is ipsilateral for the sternomastoid, but contralateral for the trapezius. The function of the sternomastoid in turning the head to the opposite side may explain this arrangement. If this pattern of cortical control is overlooked, a unilateral lesion may be misinterpreted as bilateral. In an epileptiform fit affecting one side, the head turns to that side.

The spinal accessory nerve may be damaged during excision of lymph glands from the posterior triangle or, less commonly, in fracture of the cranial base. Such lower motor neuron lesions result in paralysis and atrophy of the affected muscles.

THE VAGUS (X) AND GLOSSOPHARYNGEAL (IX) NERVES

The *vagus and glossopharyngeal nerves* are so closely alike in their nuclear origins and functional components that they are to be considered together, and the cranial root of accessory nerve is included with the vagus. They are predominantly visceral, with only a minor somatic content. Their visceral components may be summarized as follows:

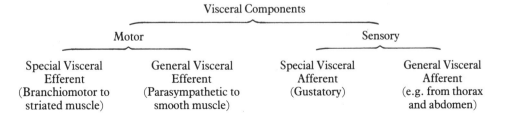

Visceral Components			
Motor		Sensory	
Special Visceral Efferent (Branchiomotor to striated muscle)	General Visceral Efferent (Parasympathetic to smooth muscle)	Special Visceral Afferent (Gustatory)	General Visceral Afferent (e.g. from thorax and abdomen)

Motor components

1. *Branchiomotor* fibres arise in the *nucleus ambiguus*, a longitudinal column of motor neurons in the medulla. From its embryonic position (*Fig.* 6.1B) it is displaced ventrolaterally to lie dorsomedial to the inferior olivary nucleus. This explains the dorsal looping of its fibres before they curve laterally to join other components (*Fig.* 6.6). Most of the output enters the vagus, either directly or via the cranial root of the accessory; it supplies muscles of the soft palate (except tensor palati which is supplied by the fifth nerve), pharynx, larynx and striated muscle of the upper oesophagus. The contribution to the glossopharyngeal nerve is small, supplying only the stylopharyngeus. The nucleus ambiguus has been termed the 'nucleus of phonation and deglutition'; these functions are impaired when it is damaged.

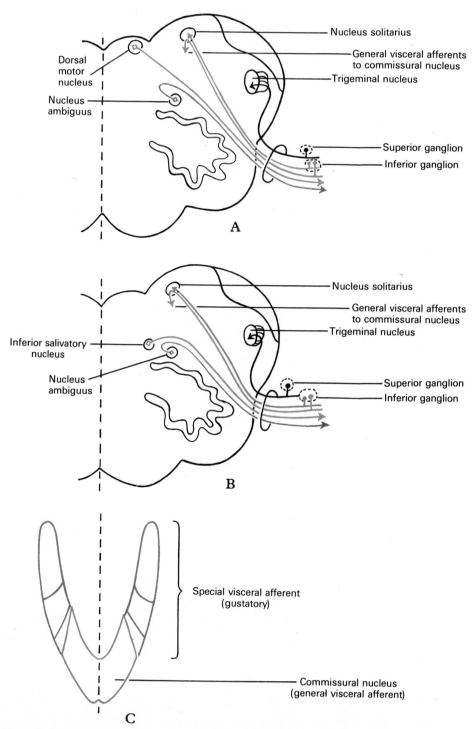

Fig. 6.6 Components of the vagus (A) and glossopharyngeal (B) nerves (C) Nucleus solitarius. Green: general visceral afferent and efferent (parasympathetic). Blue: special visceral efferent (branchiomotor). Red: special visceral afferent (gustatory). Black: general somatic afferent.

Cortical control of each nucleus ambiguus is bilateral; after a unilateral 'stroke' damaging the internal capsule the patient can still phonate and swallow. A cortical lesion in the 'dominant' hemisphere may affect language and speech centres. Reflex connexions from sensory vagal nuclei are involved in coughing and vomiting; those from the trigeminal sensory nucleus are tested by the 'gag reflex', excited by touching the soft palate or pharynx.

2. *Parasympathetic components.*
   a. The largest parasympathetic nucleus is the *dorsal vagal motor nucleus*, a column of small nerve cells extending from the vagal triangle in the rhomboid fossa into the grey matter around the central canal of the closed part of the medulla. It is *visceromotor* to involuntary muscle in the bronchi, heart, oesophagus, stomach, small intestine and the proximal two-thirds of the colon. So-called 'vital centres' for cardiac and respiratory control, and reflex centres for swallowing and vomiting, are located in the fourth ventricle's floor. Vagal parasympathetic supply is also *secretomotor* to the gastrointestinal glands and pancreas; the fibres are preganglionic, and synapse in small ganglia and plexuses near or in the walls of viscera. The nucleus receives afferents from the hypothalamus, rhinencephalon, autonomic reticular centres in the brainstem and gustatory impulses from the nucleus solitarius.
   b. *The inferior salivatory nucleus* is the source of parasympathetic fibres in the glossopharyngeal nerve to the otic ganglion, from which postganglionic fibres are *secretomotor* and *vasomotor* to the parotid gland. In addition to supranuclear influences from the hypothalamus and rhinencephalon, reflex connexions from the nucleus solitarius (taste) and the trigeminal sensory nucleus (intra-oral general stimuli) induce salivation.

Sensory components

The *nucleus solitarius* receives gustatory (special visceral) afferents from the facial, glossopharyngeal and vagus, their nuclear terminations being in a rostrocaudal sequence of decreasing size (*Figs. 6.3, 6.6*). The most caudal region receives general visceral afferents: it reaches the midline in the closed part of medulla, and is sometimes termed the '*commissural nucleus*'. The tract containing all these afferent fibres is surrounded by the nucleus, and hence is obvious in Weigert-stained sections. The cell bodies of all the primary visceral afferent neurons are in the inferior glossopharyngeal and vagal ganglia.

1. *Special visceral afferents (gustatory)* in the glossopharyngeal nerve supply the posterior third of the tongue. The vagal content of such fibres is small and limited to the epiglottic region.
2. *General visceral afferents* are received from all thoracic and abdominal viscera. Baroreceptors in the carotid sinus monitor changes in blood pressure and chemoreceptors in the carotid body respond to fluctuations of oxygen tension in the blood: these impulses travel in the glossopharyngeal nerve, and vagal fibres serve similar receptors in the aortic arch.

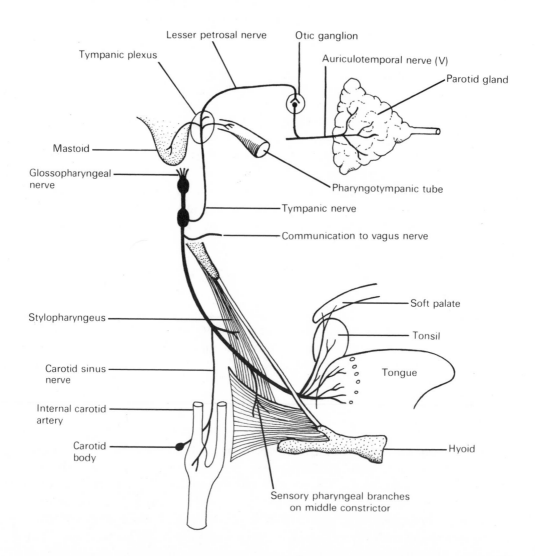

Fig. 6.7 Distribution of the right glossopharyngeal nerve. (After Grant J. C. B. (1949) *Atlas of Anatomy.* London, Baillière Tindall.)

3. *General somatic afferents* have the cell bodies of primary sensory neurons in the superior ganglia of the ninth and tenth nerves. Their dendrites are in the vagal auricular and glossopharyngeal tympanic branches; they also conduct impulses of touch and pain in the ninth and tenth nerves from the pharynx and the posterior third of the tongue. When these afferents reach the medulla they enter the *spinal trigeminal nucleus*.

Distribution of the glossopharyngeal nerve (*Fig.* 6.7)

The *tympanic nerve* supplies sensory fibres via the tympanic plexus to the middle ear, mastoid air cells and pharyngotympanic tube. Parasympathetic fibres travel via the *lesser petrosal nerve* to the otic ganglion, synapse there and join the mandibular auriculo-temporal branch of the trigeminal to supply secretomotor and vasomotor fibres to the parotid gland. The *carotid nerve* carries afferent fibres from the carotid sinus and body. *Pharyngeal nerves* share in the pharyngeal plexus and supply the pharynx, soft palate, tonsil and posterior third of the tongue. The *motor supply* is to the stylopharyngeus muscle.

Distribution of the vagus nerve (*Fig.* 6.8)

Cervical

In the jugular foramen a *meningeal nerve* branches off to supply the dura mater in the posterior cranial fossa. An *auricular* branch supplies the exterior of the ear drum, the posterior wall of the external auditory meatus and the cranial surface of the auricle. The *pharyngeal nerve(s)* form a plexus with glossopharyngeal and sympathetic fibres. The motor supply to pharynx and larynx is derived from the cranial accessory nerve. The *superior laryngeal nerve* has two branches: the *internal laryngeal nerve* pierces the thyrohyoid membrane and is sensory to the mucosa of pharynx and larynx from the level of the epiglottis to the vocal folds; the *external laryngeal nerve* is motor to the crico-thyroid. The *recurrent laryngeal nerves* loop under the subclavian artery (right) and aortic arch (left) and are motor to all intrinsic laryngeal muscles except the cricothyroid; they are also sensory to the mucosa of larynx and pharynx below the level of the vocal folds. The *cardiac nerves* arise in the neck and descend to the cardiac plexuses.

Thoracic

The *bronchial and pulmonary nerves* form a plexus with sympathetic fibres, mainly behind the root of each lung, to supply the smooth muscle and glands of the bronchial tree, the pulmonary blood vessels and the visceral and mediastinal pleura. Afferent fibres are essential to respiratory reflexes. Both vagi contribute motor and sensory fibres to the *oesophageal plexus*, joined by sympathetic fibres from the greater splanchnic nerves. Branches from the left vagus to the aortic arch and from the right vagus to the brachiocephalic artery serve *baroreceptors* and *chemoreceptors*.

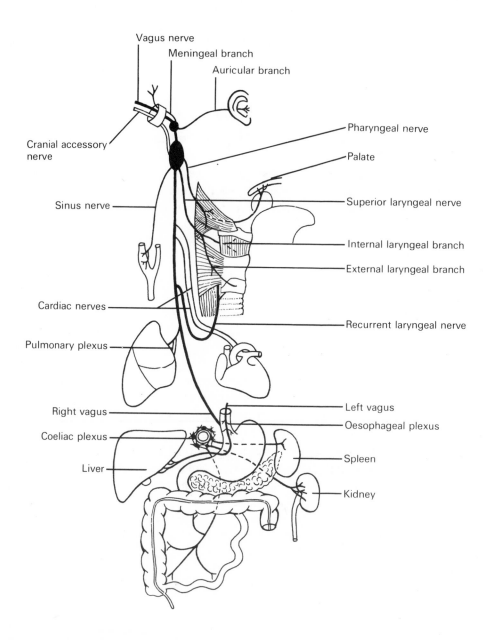

Fig. 6.8 Distribution of the right vagus nerve. (After Grant J. C. B. (1949) *Atlas of Anatomy*. London, Baillière Tindall.)

Abdominal

The anterior and posterior trunks of the vagus descend from the oesophageal plexus as *gastric nerves* supplying the corresponding surfaces of the stomach. The anterior gastric distribution extends through the lesser omentum to the liver. The posterior trunk of the vagus, in addition to its gastric branches, sends rami to the *coeliac, superior and inferior mesenteric plexuses*, distributed along these arteries to the gastrointestinal tract as far as the mid-transverse colon, and to the liver, pancreas, spleen, kidneys and suprarenal glands.

APPLIED ANATOMY

Unilateral supranuclear lesions rarely cause motor disturbance, since the glosso-pharyngeal and vagal nuclei have a bilateral cortical innervation. A cortical lesion may affect the speech and language centres, present in the 'dominant' hemisphere. Because the larynx and pharynx have bilateral cortical representation, a unilateral lesion of their corticobulbar fibres may pass unnoticed; if subsequently similar fibres in the internal capsule on the *opposite* side are damaged, speech, chewing and swallowing become impossible – a condition known as 'pseudobulbar palsy'. Bilateral degenerative or demyelinating disease causes difficulty in speaking (dysarthria) and swallowing (dysphagia) and there is a rapid heart beat (tachycardia).

The recurrent layngeal nerve is close to the inferior thyroid artery and is at risk when this vessel is ligated during thyroidectomy, or it may be subjected to traction during operation on a very large thyroid. A bilateral lesion is particularly serious, because paralysis of the vocal cord abductors ensues, and the only unaffected muscle, the cricothyroid, tenses them. If carcinoma of the lung spreads to tracheobronchial glands on the left side, the nerve may be compressed, making the voice hoarse.

Vagotomy, or abdominal division of the vagus nerves, is performed to reduce gastric acidity in duodenal ulceration; relative overaction of the sympathetic supply then causes pyloric spasm, which is rectified either by cutting the sphincter (pyloroplasty) or by anastomosing the stomach to the jejunum (gastrojejeunostomy). Sectioning of the nerves just above the cardia (truncal vagotomy) often leads to unpleasant gastro-intestinal sequelae. Selective vagotomy of particular gastric branches is hence favoured by some surgeons.

THE VESTIBULOCOCHLEAR (VIII) NERVE

The *vestibulocochlear nerve* transmits impulses from the internal ear and has two functional components: the vestibular nerve serves equilibration, and the cochlear is the nerve of hearing. Emerging from the internal auditory meatus, the nerve enters the brainstem in the lateral groove between the pons and medulla, the cochlear division being dorsal to the vestibular. This region is often described as the cerebellopontine angle.

The vestibular nerve

The vestibular part of the inner ear comprises three *semicircular canals* opening into the *utricle*, which connects with the *saccule*, itself continuous with the *cochlear duct* via the *ductus reuniens* (*Fig. 6.9*). This *membranous labyrinth* is filled with endolymph and separated from its surrounding osseous labyrinth by perilymph. The semicircular canals are at right angles to one another, and at one end of each a dilatation, or *ampulla*, contains a ridge, or *crista*, of neuroepithelial hair cells covered by a gelatinous *cupola*. Movements of the head displace the endolymph and cupola, and this stimulates the hair cells. The utricle and saccule have similar sensory epithelium in their *maculae*, the hair cells of which are in contact with an *otolithic membrane* formed of gelatinous material in which calcareous otoliths or particles are embedded.

The vestibular nerve consists of the central fibres of bipolar cells in the *vestibular ganglion*, in the depths of the internal auditory meatus. The shorter peripheral fibres pass either to the cristae of the semicircular canals (*kinetic labyrinth*), concerned with head *movements* or to the maculae of the utricle and saccule (*static labyrinth*), concerned with head *position*. Entering the medulla ventral to the inferior cerebellar peduncle, the central fibres pass to the *vestibular nuclei*, in the floor of the fourth ventricle's lateral angle; some fibres bypass these nuclei to enter the cerebellum directly via its inferior peduncle, indicating the intimate interrelationship, both functional and phylogenetic, between labyrinth and cerebellum.

The four vestibular nuclei are the lateral (Deiter's nucleus), superior, medial and inferior (*Fig. 6.10*); they influence the cerebellum, spinal cord and oculogyric nuclei, and have cortical connexions. The cerebellar connexions are reciprocal; the cerebellum projects to all the vestibular nuclei. The archecerebellum is concerned with equilibration and the paleocerebellum with muscle tone. The archecerebellum receives input from the superior, medial and inferior vestibular nuclei and directly from the vestibular nerve.

Paths to the spinal cord are via the vestibulospinal and reticulospinal tracts. The *ventrolateral vestibulospinal tract* starts in the lateral vestibular (Deiter's) nucleus and descends throughout the ventral white column, synapsing with α and γ motor neurons. Fibres from the medial and inferior vestibular nuclei of both sides descend in the *medial longitudinal fasciculus* as a *medial vestibulospinal tract* in the cervical cord, influencing tone in the neck muscles and effecting balancing movements in the upper limbs. The *reticulospinal* tracts also affect muscle tone, and are also involved in bodily reactions to vestibular disturbance, as in sea-sickness.

In the *brainstem*, the vestibular nuclei connect with the oculogyric (III, IV, VI) nuclei via the *medial longitudinal fasciculus*, and reciprocally with the *reticular formation*. This fasciculus extends bilaterally throughout the brainstem, flanking the midline. Ascending fibres in it from the superior vestibular nucleus are ipsilateral, those from the lateral and inferior nuclei are contralateral, and those from the medial nucleus are bilateral (*Fig. 6.10*). These connexions co-ordinate movements of the head and eyes, influenced by input from the kinetic labyrinth. There are caudal connexions with the accessory nerve's spinal root. The medial longitudinal fasciculus also mediates co-ordination between the oculogyric nuclei, essential to binocular vision. A 'centre for lateral gaze' in or near the para-abducent nucleus co-ordinates the innervation of the

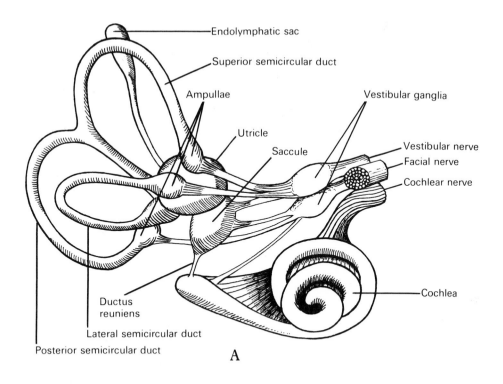

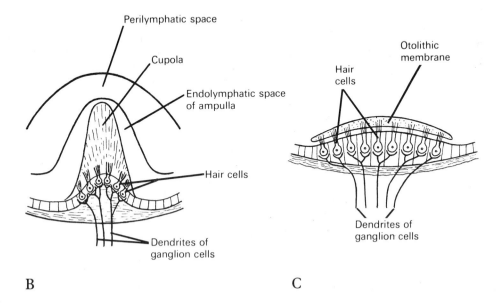

Fig. 6.9 Distribution of the vestibulocochlear nerve to (A) the membranous labyrinth, (B) the sensory apparatus of the utricle and (C) a semicircular duct.

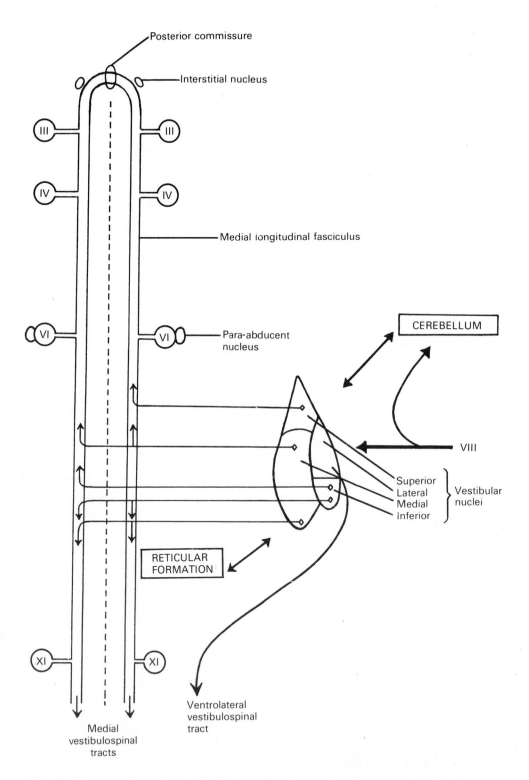

Fig. 6.10 Connexions of the medial longitudinal fasciculi and vestibular nuclei.

lateral rectus (supplied by the abducent nerve) with that of the contralateral medial rectus (supplied by the oculomotor nerve). The two medial longitudinal fasciculi are interconnected via the posterior commissure. The fasciculi are also a general association bundle between brainstem motor nuclei, providing connexions between the oculomotor and facial nuclei co-ordinating movement of the eyelids, or between the nucleus ambiguus, fifth, seventh and twelfth nerves in speech, mastication and swallowing. Extrapyramidal influences may reach the motor nuclei via the interstitial nucleus (of Cajal).

Vestibular *cortical connexions* are uncertain: vestibular activity elicits responses from the ventral posterior nucleus of the thalamus. Stimulation of the human superior temporal gyrus evokes vertigo. In monkeys the primary cortical connexion appears to be in the lower part of the postcentral gyrus.

APPLIED ANATOMY

Vestibular function may be tested by the experimental induction of *nystagmus*, that is rhythmic ocular movements, the eyes rotating rapidly in one direction and returning more slowly. Nystagmus may be physiological or pathological. In the *rotatory test* a patient is spun on a vertical axis about ten times. When body rotation is arrested suddenly, fluid in the semicircular canals continues to move, evoking impulses in the nerve; if it and its connexions are intact, nystagmus occurs. In the *caloric test,* warm or cold water, instilled into the external auditory meatus, causes currents in the endolymph of the canals, with similar results. The subject is unable to walk along a straight line; in attempting to point at an object the arm deviates or overshoots ('past pointing').

Dysfunction is accompanied by vertigo, nausea, vomiting and nystagmus, as may occur in diseases of the labyrinth, in disabling paroxysms in *Ménière's disease*. The eighth nerve sometimes develops a primary tumour: such an *acoustic neuroma* causes deafness, vestibular disturbance and symptoms due to pressure on nerves near the cerebello-pontine angle. The medial longitudinal fasciculus is peculiarly susceptible to demyelination in *disseminated sclerosis*.

The cochlear nerve

The auditory pathways mediate highly discriminative perception of sound at cortical level, and also subcortical reflex reactions to sound.

The *cochlear* part of the labyrinth is a spiral of two and a half turns, divided into three channels by the *basilar and vestibular membranes*, forming the *scala vestibuli, scala tympani* and *cochlear duct* (*Fig.* 6.11). The stapes fit in an oval window at the base of the scala vestibuli; a round window is closed by a flexible membrane at the base of the scala tympani. At the apex of the bony core, or *modiolus*, the scalae vestibuli and tympani are in continuity by a narrow passage, the *helicotrema*.

The *spiral organ* (of Corti) (*Fig.* 6.11) is an auditory transducer; its *receptor hair cells* are arranged in an inner row and three outer rows, supported on a basilar membrane by

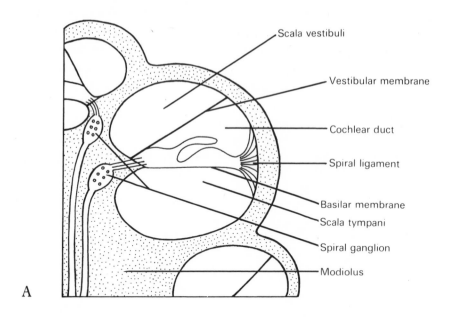

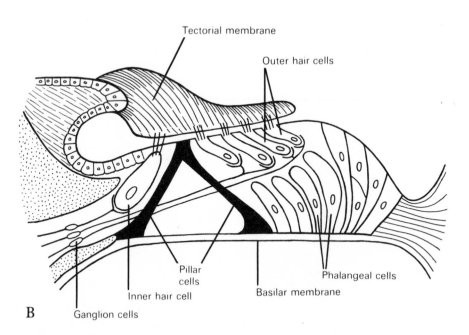

Fig. 6.11 Structure of the cochlea. (A) Section through part of the cochlea. (B) The spiral organ of Corti.

phalangeal cells and attached by their hair processes to an overlying *tectorial membrane*. The basilar membrane is not taut and its mobility varies along the cochlea; it is narrowest and most rigid at the cochlear base, widest and slackest at the apex. Stapedial movement transmits sound waves to perilymph in the scala vestibuli, displacing the basilar membrane and bending hair cells attached to the relatively immobile tectorial membrane.

The cochlear nerve consists of the central processes of bipolar cells in the *spiral ganglion*, located in the modiolus. Reaching the medulla, the nerve divides into a dorsal and a ventral root. The former curves over the inferior cerebellar peduncle to the *dorsal cochlear nucleus*, which forms a small eminence, the *acoustic tubercle*, on the upper surface of the peduncle in the floor of the lateral recess of the fourth ventricle. The ventral root ends in the *ventral cochlear nucleus* on the inferior aspect of the peduncle. There is tonotopic localization throughout the auditory system; high frequencies are received at the base of the cochlea, low frequencies at the apex. Similarly, neuron bodies in the nuclei responding to high frequencies are dorsal, while those responding to low frequencies are ventral. Neuronal connexions are highly discrete in the ventral nucleus; in the dorsal nucleus the afferents synapse with a larger number of cells, permitting summation and facilitation, significant in reflex responses. The central projections of both nuclei are shown in *Fig*. 6.12.

From the ventral cochlear nucleus fibres decussate in the *trapezoid body* to reach the contralateral *superior olivary nucleus*, where some synapse; others have already synapsed in the ipsilateral olivary nucleus, and some ascend ipsilaterally. Fibres from the dorsal nucleus cross more superficially and make similar connexions, and then join efferents of the ventral nucleus to ascend in the *lateral lemniscus*, which contains secondary *and* tertiary neurons. In the small *nucleus of the lateral lemniscus* other synapses occur. Ascending fibres relay in the *inferior colliculus*, and then traverse the inferior brachium to the *medial geniculate body*. Through the *auditory radiation* the path reaches the *auditory cortex* of the temporal lobe (Brodmann areas 41, 42), deep in the lateral fissure (transverse temporal gyri) and extending slightly onto the external surface. A tonotopic pattern is maintained, low frequency sounds being appreciated anteriorly, high frequency posteriorly, in the auditory area. Secondary cochlear paths are crossed and uncrossed; fibres from one side ascend in both lemnisci, with a commissure between the inferior colliculi. Thus a unilateral cortical lesion, or damage to one lateral lemniscus, affects hearing on both sides. Connexions between the auditory paths and the reticular formation are involved in reflex arousal.

Descending fibres exist in the auditory pathways, some projecting from the cortex to the medial geniculate body and inferior colliculus. Others descend from the inferior colliculus to cochlear nuclei, concerned with 'neural sharpening' and increased qualitative perception. The *olivocochlear bundle* extends from the superior olivary nucleus through the cochlear nerve to the spiral organ (of Corti), and can suppress transmission of acoustic stimuli. To some degree auditory stimuli can be ignored or selected; a mother may sleep despite traffic noise, yet awake if her child cries. We need not attend closely to 'background music'. Listening to radio and watching television show differences between the 'control' mechanisms on the auditory and the more compulsive ('hypnotic') visual inputs.

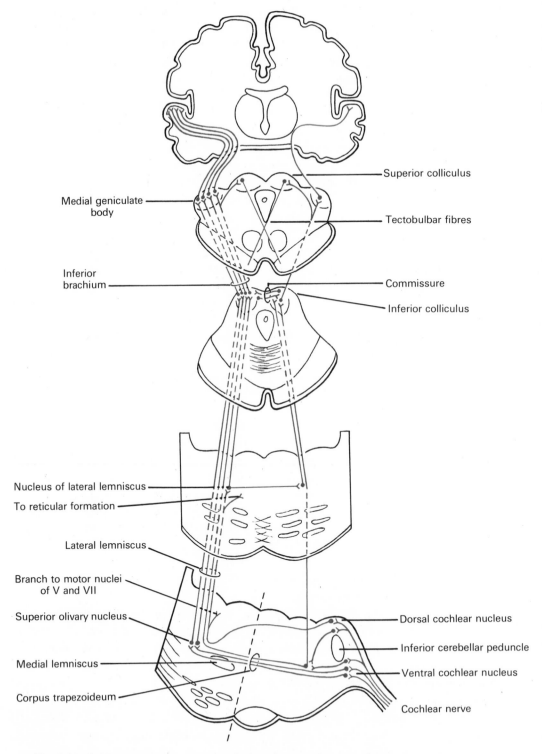

Fig. 6.12 Auditory pathways. The lowest section, at the pontomedullary junction, is oblique, through the pons on the left and the medulla on the right.

Auditory reflexes

The ears, head and eyes are turned automatically towards an unexpected sound, the reflexes mediated in part from the inferior to the superior colliculus, and thence by tectobulbar and tectospinal tracts. A loud noise may 'startle'; extreme percussion of a stun grenade produces a transient 'freeze', probably through auditory projection to the reticular formation. Effects via the ascending reticular system in arousal from sleep, or its prevention, are commonplace. Connexions from the superior olivary nucleus to the trigeminal motor nucleus evoke reflex contractions in tensor tympani and, via the facial nerve, in stapedius, which dampen excessive vibrations in the tympanic membrane and stapes due to very loud noise.

APPLIED ANATOMY

It is necessary to determine whether deafness is due to damage in the middle ear, or in the nerve and its receptors. In middle ear disease, if the nerve is intact, the sound of a tuning fork applied to the mastoid process (bone conduction) is louder than if held near the external ear (air conduction). Cochlear damage often produces permanent tinnitus. The nerve may be damaged in head injuries, or be the site of a primary tumour (acoustic neuroma).

THE FACIAL (VII) NERVE

The *facial nerve* emerges at the lower pontine border in two parts or 'roots', a large *motor root*, and a smaller '*sensory*' *root* (*Fig.* 6.13). The latter contains not only afferent fibres but also an efferent (parasympathetic) component, and is more aptly termed '*nervus intermedius*', being between the facial motor root and the vestibulocochlear nerve in the cerebellopontine angle. Since it supplies the second branchial arch, its morphological components are mostly visceral, its somatic sensory input small.

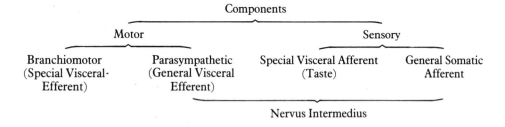

Motor components

1. *Branchiomotor*. The *motor nucleus* is in the caudal pontine tegmentum, rostral to the nucleus ambiguus and in the same special visceral efferent 'column'. Evolving in the floor of the fourth ventricle, it has migrated ventrolaterally through 'neurobiotaxis', whereby functionally associated centres are said to become approximated. Thus the nucleus of VII moves towards that of V, and that of VI towards the medial

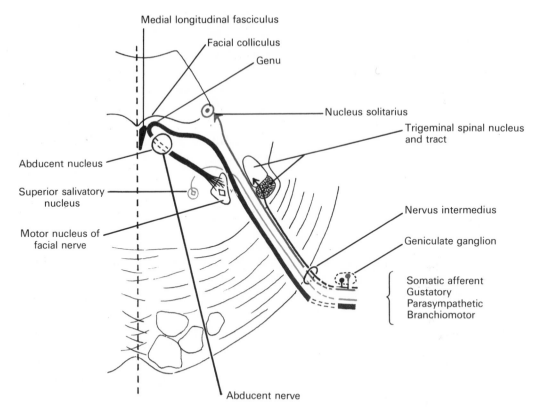

Fig. 6.13 Components of the facial nerve in the pons. Blue: special visceral efferent (branchiomotor). Green: general visceral efferent (parasympathetic). Red: special visceral afferent (gustatory). Black: general somatic afferent.

longitudinal fasciculus. This may explain the complex route of the facial efferent fibres, which loop dorsally over the abducent nucleus, producing the *facial colliculus*, and then arch ventrally between the nucleus of origin and the trigeminal spinal nucleus to reach the surface. These fibres supply the facial muscles, plus platysma, stylohyoid, posterior belly of digastric and stapedius. Cortical control of lower facial muscles is strictly contralateral, but the upper face (orbicularis oculi and frontalis) has bilateral cortical innervation, a useful fact in distinguishing between upper and lower motor neuron lesions. There is also a supranuclear influence from subcortical centres concerned with emotion: when this is lost in Parkinson's disease the so-called 'mask-like facies' ensues.

There are reflex connexions. In the corneal reflex, eyelids close (VII) in response to corneal irritation (V). Loud noise causes reflex contraction of stapedius (VII) via afferents from the superior olivary nucleus (VIII). Tectobulbar fibres from superior colliculus mediate a protective blink reflex and narrowing of the palpebral fissure in response to bright light

2. *Parasympathetic.* General visceral efferent fibres from cells in a *superior salivatory nucleus* leave in the nervus intermedius. These preganglionic secretomotor and

vasomotor fibres relay in ganglia to supply the submandibular and sublingual salivary glands and the palatine and lacrimal glands. Fibres reach the pterygopalatine ganglion via the greater petrosal nerve, and the submandibular ganglion via the chorda tympani (*Fig.* 6.14). A supranuclear input from the hypothalamus via the *dorsal longitudinal fasciculus* (not to be confused with the medial longitudinal fasciculus) mediates emotional lacrimation, and olfactory connexions may initiate salivation. Reflex salivation is also evoked by the taste of food (via the nucleus solitarius). Oral irritation causes salivation, and in the eye produces lacrimation: in each case afferent impulses traverse the trigeminal sensory nucleus.

Sensory components

The afferent fibres are mostly visceral (taste), and the somatic are few. All primary sensory neurons have their unipolar cell bodies in the *geniculate ganglion*, at the bend or *genu* of the facial nerve in the petrous wall of the middle ear.

1. *Special Visceral Afferent* (Taste). The dendrites are largely in the anterior two-thirds of the tongue, centripetal fibres in the chorda tympani. Afferents from the soft palate and palatal arches traverse the greater petrosal nerve. Centripetal axons from the geniculate ganglion traverse the nervus intermedius to enter the rostral part of the *nucleus solitarius* (*Fig.* 6.6); gustatory impulses pass from this to the hypothalamus and ventral posterior thalamic nucleus, and thence to the 'face region' of the sensory cortex. Reflex connexions to salivatory nuclei have been mentioned; connexions with the dorsal vagal motor nucleus mediate their effects on gastric secretion and gastrointestinal motility.

2. *General Somatic Afferent*. Some fibres from the external auditory meatus, tympanic membrane and postaural skin join the facial nerve via the vagal auricular branch, traversing the nervus intermedius to end (like similar fibres in glossopharyngeal and vagus nerves) in the *spinal nucleus of the trigeminal nerve*. The facial nerve is *not* sensory to the face.

Course and distribution of the facial nerve

This abbreviated account is supplemented by *Fig.* 6.14. The motor root and nervus intermedius join in the internal auditory meatus, pierce its lateral wall and enter the *facial canal*, where the nerve runs anterolaterally above and between the cochlea and the vestibule. At its *genu* (site of the geniculate ganglion) it turns posteriorly in the middle ear's medial wall and then downwards in the medial wall of the mastoid aditus to exit through the *stylomastoid foramen*. Passing anterolaterally it finally enters the parotid gland, subdividing into terminal branches.

Leaving the geniculate ganglion, the *greater petrosal nerve* enters the middle cranial fossa, is joined at the foramen lacerum by the deep petrosal nerve (sympathetic fibres from internal carotid plexus) to form the *nerve of the pterygoid canal*, which goes to

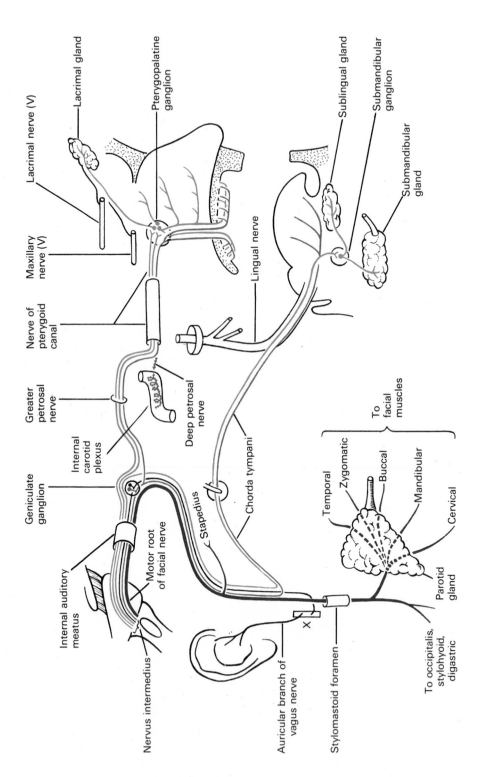

Fig. 6.14 The course and distribution of components of the facial nerve. Blue: branchiomotor. Green: parasympathetic efferent. Beaded red line from internal carotid plexus: sympathetic. Red: afferent gustatory. Black: general somatic afferent.

the pterygopalatine ganglion. The *nerve to stapedius* branches off in the facial canal. A *communicating branch* joins the auricular branch of the vagus. The *chorda tympani* leaves the facial nerve above the stylomastoid foramen, ascends to cross the tympanic membrane and leaves the middle ear via the petrotympanic fissure to join the lingual nerve (V), which distributes its taste fibres to the anterior two-thirds of the tongue, and its preganglionic fibres to the *submandibular ganglion*. As the facial nerve leaves the stylomastoid foramen, the *posterior auricular nerve* branches to supply the occipitalis and posterior auricular muscles, and a *digastric* branch supplies the posterior belly of the digastric and stylohyoid muscles; it then divides into *terminal branches* – temporal, zygomatic, buccal, mandibular and cervical – to the *facial muscles*.

APPLIED ANATOMY

Supranuclear lesions are usually part of a hemiplegia due to a cerebrovascular accident; only the muscles below the palpebral fissures are completely paralysed; the patient can still close the eyelids and wrinkle the forehead. In cortical or capsular lesions, voluntary and emotional facial activity may be dissociated: the patient can still smile if amused but be unable to 'show his teeth' on demand. By contrast, the retention of voluntary movement but loss of spontaneous emotional expression characterizes Parkinson's disease.

The commonest of *infranuclear* lesions is *Bell's palsy*, thought to be of viral origin, in which oedema compresses the nerve within its canal. It may be damaged in *fracture* of the cranial base, affected by *inflammation of the middle ear* and mastoid air cells, or compressed in the cerebellopontine angle by an *acoustic neuroma*; the ipsilateral upper and lower facial muscles are all paralysed. Inability to close the eyelids may lead to corneal ulceration, especially if reflex lacrimation is also lost.

The extent of loss in lower motor neuron lesions depends on the level of injury. If this is proximal to the geniculate ganglion, taste is lost in the anterior two-thirds of the tongue and secretion from the submandibular, sublingual and lacrimal glands is impaired. *Hyperacusis* (increased sound perception) is due to paralysis of stapedius. The prognosis is usually good in more distal lesions; in lesions proximal to geniculate ganglion, however, sensory regeneration is poor and salivatory parasympathetic fibres may be misdirected into the lacrimal gland, producing 'crocodile tears' in response to the smell or taste of food.

If *herpes zoster* affects the geniculate ganglion, vesicles appear on the pinna and sometimes on the soft palate and tongue.

THE ABDUCENT (VI), TROCHLEAR (IV) AND OCULOMOTOR (III) NERVES

These three nerves are interrelated anatomically in oculogyric function, and will be considered together. Their nuclei of origin are all near the medial longitudinal fasciculus, and connected with it. Each nerve contains general somatic efferent fibres; the oculomotor nerve also has a parasympathetic component. The nerves all traverse the cavernous sinus and superior orbital fissure as shown in *Fig.* 6.15.

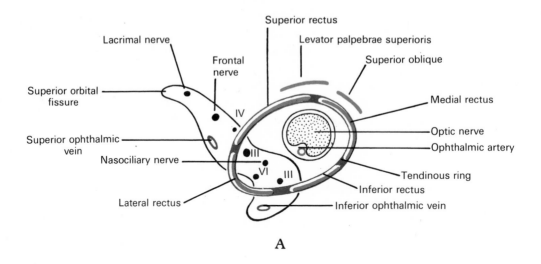

A

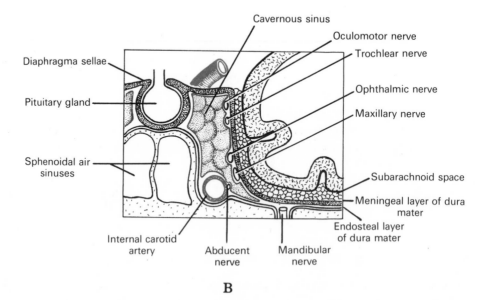

B

Fig. 6.15 Relationships of nerves in the superior orbital fissure (A) and cavernous sinus (B).

The abducent nerve

The abducent nucleus (*Fig.* 6.13) adjoins the facial colliculus at the pontine level of the fourth ventricle's floor, where motor fibres of the facial nerve loop round it. Abducent fibres descend ventrally to leave between lower pontine border and pyramid. They supply the lateral rectus. Near the main nucleus is a group of smaller cells, the *para-abducent nucleus*, the 'centre for lateral gaze', which probably co-ordinates activity between the ipsilateral lateral rectus and the contralateral medial rectus (via the medial longitudinal fasciculus and the oculomotor nucleus).

The nerve pierces the 'inner layer' of dura mater at the dorsum sellae and ascends to cross the apex of the petrous temporal bone, here angled forward lateral to the internal carotid artery in the cavernous sinus. It enters the orbit by the superior orbital fissure within the common annular tendon of the recti (*Fig.* 6.15A).

The trochlear nerve

The trochlear nucleus is in the ventral periaqueductal mesencephalic grey matter at the level of the inferior colliculus (*Fig.* 6.16). It supplies the superior oblique muscle. It has three singular features: it is the most slender cranial nerve, it decussates before emerging, and it emerges on the dorsal aspect. Its emergence is near the midline, through the superior medullary velum just caudal to the inferior colliculus. It curves round the cerebral peduncle, passes between the posterior cerebral and superior

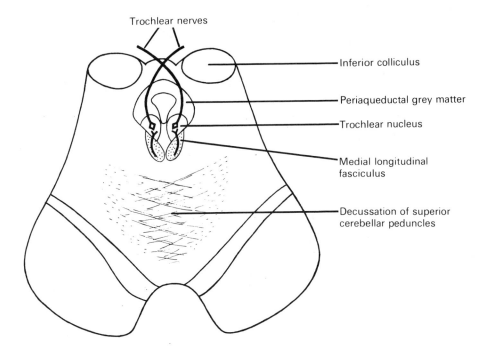

Fig. 6.16 Origin of trochlear nerves in the midbrain.

cerebellar arteries, pierces the 'inner layer' of dura mater just below the tentorial margin, and enters the lateral wall of the cavernous sinus, passing forward into the orbit via the superior orbital fissure, outside the annular tendon (*Fig.* 6.15A).

The oculomotor nerve

The oculomotor nerve contains *somatic efferent* fibres for all the extra-ocular muscles except the superior oblique and the lateral rectus. It also contains *parasympathetic efferents* to the sphincter pupillae and ciliary muscle; it receives postganglionic sympathetic fibres from the internal carotid plexus and distributes them to these two intra-ocular muscles. Its terminal branches collect proprioceptive afferents from the ocular muscles, which are transferred by communicating rami to trigeminal branches in the orbit or cavernous sinus. Ocular muscle fibres are thin and their motor units small, and in man the muscle spindles are numerous, probably to ensure accurate co-ordination of ocular movement.

From its nucleus the nerve traverses the red nucleus and substantia nigra to emerge in the interpeduncular fossa (*Fig.* 6.17), where it passes between the posterior cerebral and superior cerebellar arteries, pierces the 'inner layer' of dura mater lateral to the posterior clinoid process to enter the lateral wall of the cavernous sinus. It traverses the superior

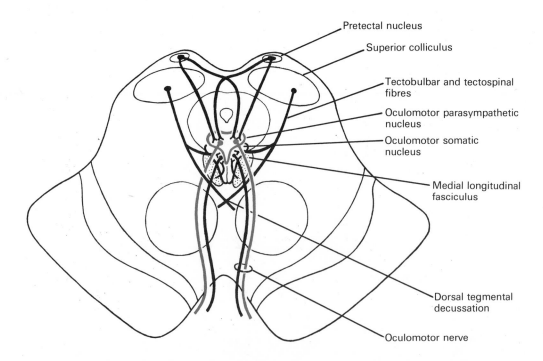

Fig. 6.17 Oculomotor nuclei and their connexions in the midbrain. Oculomotor components shown in black are somatic efferents, those in green are parasympathetic efferents from the Edinger-Westphal nucleus.

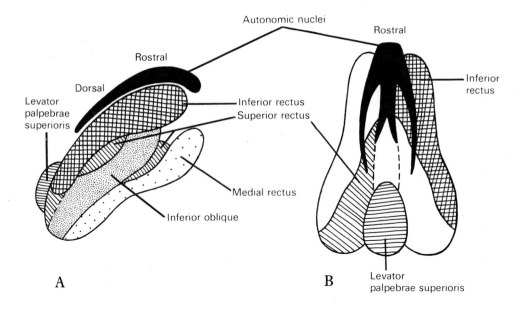

Fig. 6.18 The constituent parts of the oculomotor nucleus and their distribution in the monkey. (A) Right lateral aspect. (B) Dorsal aspect. (From Warwick R. (1953) *J. Comp. Neurol.* **98**, 480, reproduced by kind permission of the author and publisher.)

orbital fissure and annular tendon in superior and inferior divisions (*Fig.* 6.15A), the former supplying the superior rectus and levator palpebrae superioris, the latter supplying the medial and inferior recti and the inferior oblique. The branch to the inferior oblique transfers parasympathetic and sympathetic fibres to the ciliary ganglion.

The oculomotor nerve arises from a *nuclear complex*, ventral in the periaqueductal grey matter at superior collicular level, and flanked by the medial longitudinal fasciculi and tectobulbar tracts (*Fig.* 6.17). This nuclear complex has two components:

1. The *general somatic efferent* component is a series of sub-nuclei described by Warwick (1953) (*Fig.* 6.18). These are paired except for a *caudal central nucleus* supplying the levatores palpebrae superiores. Three lateral nuclei innervate the inferior rectus, inferior oblique and medial rectus, medial to which is a nucleus for the superior rectus.
2. *The parasympathetic* (general visceral efferent) component is also known as the *Edinger-Westphal nucleus*. It is dorsal to the somatic nuclei and its neurons relay in the ciliary ganglion, whence short ciliary nerves supply the sphincter pupillae and ciliaris oculi.

Control of ocular movements

Many ocular movements are involuntary, some are initiated voluntarily and continued automatically, and some are purely voluntary. Such movements are all conjugate, sometimes with superimposed convergence (*see* accommodation and pupillary reflexes, p. 125).

1. *Compensatory ocular movements* maintain a constant retinal (foveal) image despite head and body movement; the mechanism is in action during walking, when the head moves up and down with each stride. If one compares the constancy of a visual image with results from a hand-held cine camera during walking, it is evident that a compensatory mechanism is continuously at work. This is provided by the vestibular apparatus, spinovestibular pathways adding proprioceptive information from the neck muscles. (The role of the cerebellum both in equilibration and in muscular co-ordination is described in the next chapter).

2. *Pursuit eye movements and automatic scanning* allow vision to 'lock on' to a moving object. A similar mechanism operates in looking out from a moving vehicle: the eyes *fix* transiently on a succession of passing objects; looking from a train may induce temporary 'railway nystagmus', which illustrates the 'fixation reflex'. Miner's nystagmus is due to persistent subconscious attempts to fix on objects, even in darkness. Locational information passes from the primary visual cortex (Brodmann area 17) to the visual association cortex (Brodmann areas 18, 19), and descending *corticotectal and corticobulbar tracts* are involved in the response, according to clinical evidence.

   Reading is complex, being an acquired skill and dependent on cortical analysis of language. During learning, the eyes scan voluntarily, but when the ability is fully developed, scanning becomes largely reflex.

3. *Voluntary scanning* is the ability to examine an area in the visual field and to locate particular features. The frontal eye field (Brodmann area 8) co-ordinates these movements (*see* Applied Anatomy). Head movements often accompany those of the eyes.

   The *medial longitudinal fasciculus* transmits vestibular information to the oculogyric nuclei. It provides nuclear interconnexions and is linked to the para-abducent nucleus, the 'centre for lateral gaze'. The *interstitial nucleus* (of Cajal) provides a link with extrapyramidal neurons, perhaps principally in movements in the vertical plane, such as compensatory eye movements during walking.

   The *superior colliculus* appears to integrate reflex movements of the eyes, head and body in response to visual and acoustic stimuli. Ocular movements follow its experimental stimulation. A pineal tumour, as it enlarges and compresses the tectum, successively causes paralysis of elevation, depression and horizontal scan. Corticotectal input is required for 'pursuit movements' and 'visual grasp reflex'. Tracing detailed links between the superior colliculus and oculogyric nuclei is difficult experimentally. The tectobulbar tracts appear to be indirect connexions through interneurons; one such route involves the interstitial nucleus.

Pupillary reflexes

Pupillary reflexes involve the accessory autonomic oculomotor nucleus (of Edinger and Westphal). In the *light reflex*, pupillary constriction is effected at subcortical level. If one eye only is stimulated, both pupils constrict, the so-called *consensual reflex*. The afferents are optic fibres which pass to both *pretectal nuclei*, crossing in the posterior commissure. Pretectal nuclei project to the autonomic (Edinger-Westphal) nucleus, from which parasympathetic efferents traverse the oculomotor nerves to ciliary ganglia, whence postganglionic fibres in short ciliary nerves innervate the sphincter pupillae muscles.

The *accommodation reflex* effects three ocular adjustments in near vision: pupillary constriction, convergence of the optic axes and increased convexity of the lens. Since this reflex entails image analysis, optic paths to the cortex must be involved. The corticocollicular path, and connexions between the superior colliculus and the accessory autonomic (Edinger-Westphal) nucleus complete the central route. The efferent path is that of the light reflex for innervation of the sphincter pupillae and ciliaris oculi, but all the extra-ocular muscles are involved in convergence, some contracting, some relaxing *pari passu*.

Like other autonomic nuclei, the Edinger-Westphal receives an input from the hypothalamus.

APPLIED ANATOMY

Every ocular movement requires co-ordinated adjustment in all the extra-ocular muscles: the actions of individual muscles are summarized in Starling's diagram (*Fig.* 6.19).

In total *oculomotor paralysis* the ophthalmoplegia is severe: the eye is directed down and outwards due to unopposed actions of the lateral rectus and superior oblique. Ptosis (drooping) of the upper lid results from paralysis of the levator palpebrae superioris. The pupil is dilated, unresponsive to direct and consensual light reflexes, and to accommodation. Since muscular innervations originate in sub-groups, partial lesions at nuclear level may occur. In an *abducent palsy* abduction is weak (the two obliques have an abductor component), and ultimately the unopposed medial rectus produces internal strabismus. In *trochlear nerve paralysis* diplopia (double vision) occurs when the eye is directed inferomedially, since the superior oblique takes part in 'down and out' movements (and medial rotation).

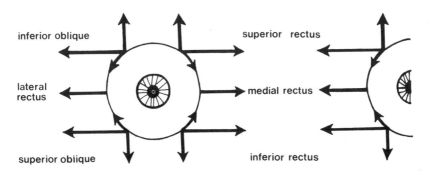

Fig. 6.19 Starling's diagram of the actions of the extrinsic ocular muscles.

The *Argyll Robertson pupil* is a phenomenon of syphilis in the central nervous system. The pupil contracts in accommodation but not to light. As noted, afferents in these two reflexes differ, and may be separately damaged. A similar phenomenon appears when a pineal tumour compresses the pretectal region.

If the *frontal eye field* is damaged, as in vascular deprivation, the patient cannot look voluntarily to the opposite side. In epileptic seizures involving this area, with cortical over-activity, the eyes are deflected contralaterally. In encephalitis, or post-encephalitic Parkinsonism, there may be *'oculogyric crises'* with strong upward deflection of the eyes' visual axes, an example of extrapyramidal dysfunction.

A pontine vascular lesion may affect the postulated *'centre for lateral gaze'* and the adjacent abducent nucleus. *Internuclear ophthalmoplegia* is due to demyelinating disease in the medial longitudinal fasciculus, often manifested by convergent or divergent squint, or by inco-ordination between the medial and lateral recti.

THE TRIGEMINAL (V) NERVE

The *trigeminal nerve* is sensory to the face, scalp, mouth, teeth, nasal cavity and air sinuses, and motor to the masticatory muscles. It is continuous with the ventral pontine surface via a large *sensory root* and, anteromedial to this, a smaller *motor root*.

Sensory components (general somatic afferent)

Most trigeminal sensory fibres have unipolar cell bodies in the *trigeminal ganglion*, in a small recess of dura mater (cavum trigeminale), near the apex of the petrous temporal bone. It differs from a dorsal root ganglion, firstly because there are no visceral afferents, and secondly because proprioceptive fibres pass through it to form a *mesencephalic tract*, with cell bodies of primary neurons in the midbrain. The three divisions, ophthalmic, maxillary and mandibular, converge on the ganglion. The motor root passes under the ganglion to the mandibular division for distribution. Cutaneous input to the trigeminal sensory nuclei includes small somatic afferent components in the facial and glossopharyngeal nerves, already described. *Trigeminal sensory nuclei form a column* throughout the brainstem, extending into the first two cervical spinal segments (*Fig.* 6.20); there is a rostrocaudal segregation of sensory modalities in this column.

The *mesencephalic nucleus*, mediating proprioception, is a slender column of *unipolar primary neurons* sited laterally in the periaqueductal grey matter of the midbrain, reaching caudally to the lateral angle of the fourth ventricle. It is flanked by input fibres, the *mesencephalic tract*. It receives afferents from neuromuscular spindles of the masticatory muscles and from the temporomandibular joint and the teeth. There is acute intra-oral proprioception, essential in chewing, controlling the force and accuracy of the bite – how rarely the tongue is bitten, and how aware one is initially of minor structural change due to dental surgery! This nucleus may also receive input from proprioceptors in the extra-ocular and facial muscles.

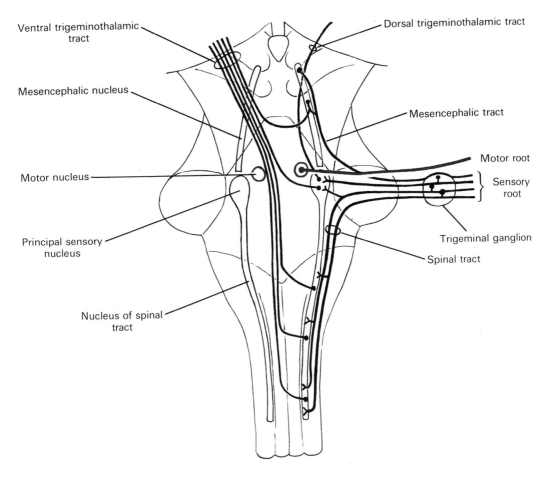

Fig. 6.20 Trigeminal nuclei and their connexions.

Other trigeminal sensory fibres traverse the basilar pons, many dividing into ascending and descending branches: the ascending fibres enter the *principal trigeminal nucleus*, which mediates discriminative touch and is homologous with the dorsal column spinal nuclei; the descending fibres, finely myelinated or non-myelinated, form the *trigeminal spinal tract*, which enters the *trigeminal spinal nucleus*, which is continuous rostrally with the principal nucleus and descends to the second cervical spinal segment to blend with the substantia gelatinosa. According to its cytoarchitecture and functions the spinal nucleus has been subdivided into a *pars rostralis* and a *pars interpolaris*, both mediating simple touch and pressure sensation, and a *pars caudalis* concerned with pain and temperature modalities. The spinal nucleus therefore corresponds to nuclei of the spinal dorsal grey horn, and has similar processing mechanisms for modulation of input. Afferents from the three trigeminal divisions rotate, bringing mandibular fibres to a dorsal position in the tract and nucleus, with maxillary fibres central and ophthalmic afferents ventral (*Fig.* 6.21). Moreover, the ophthalmic input extends to cervical level, the maxillary input terminates rostral to this, and the mandibular input does not pass

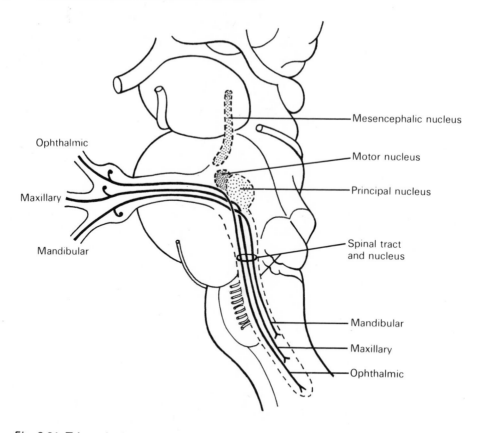

Fig. 6.21 Trigeminal nuclei from lateral aspect. Note that in the spinal nucleus the ophthalmic division is ventral and extends caudally to the cervical region; the mandibular division is dorsal and terminates at mid-medullary level. (After Brodal A. (1981) *Neurological Anatomy*. Oxford, Oxford University Press.)

caudal to mid-medullary level. This information has diagnostic and therapeutic value (*see* Applied Anatomy). The spinal tract includes components from the facial, glosso-pharyngeal and vagus nerves for general somatic sensation in the ear, tongue, pharynx and larynx.

Trigeminal *central projections* are thalamic, cerebellar and nuclear. Fibres from the spinal nucleus reach the medial *ventral posterior thalamic nucleus* via the crossed *ventral trigeminothalamic* tract sited immediately dorsal to the contralateral medial lemniscus. From the principal sensory nucleus most fibres cross, but some ascend in a smaller uncrossed dorsal trigeminothalamic tract (*Fig.* 6.20), which ascends through the dorsal pontine tegmentum to lie close to the periaqueductal grey matter in the midbrain. Cortical representation is highly specific and illustrates the functional organization of the cortex into vertical cell units, as experimentally demonstrated in regard to rats' vibrissae: each hair is apparently associated with a single 'barrel' of cells.

The mesencephalic nucleus is connected to the *cerebellum* via its superior peduncle, the spinal nucleus via the inferior peduncle.

Reflex arcs involve the trigeminal, facial and hypoglossal motor nuclei, the nucleus ambiguus and the reticular formation. An example is the corneal reflex: touching the cornea evokes impulses in the ophthalmic nerve, and reflex eyelid closure is effected via the facial nerve. Obviously nuclei controlling mastication, swallowing and phonation must also be co-ordinated. Nasal irritation provokes sneezing, which involves widespread muscular response through reticulospinal pathways. Toothache may inhibit sleep, an effect mediated via the reticular activating system.

Motor component

The *trigeminal motor nucleus* is medial to the principal sensory nucleus. It is branchiomotor to derivatives of the first branchial arch, and is distributed via the mandibular nerve to the muscles of mastication (masseter, temporalis, medial and lateral pterygoids) and to four others (tensor palati, tensor tympani, mylohyoid and the anterior belly of digastric). It receives a bilateral corticonuclear innervation; masticatory muscles act bilaterally.

Course and distribution of the trigeminal nerve (*Fig. 6.22*)

It must be noted that although the trigeminal nerve has no *intrinsic* parasympathetic component each division, in its branches, is *associated with parasympathetic ganglia*, and distributes their postganglionic fibres.

The *ophthalamic division* traverses the superior orbital fissure as frontal, lacrimal and nasociliary branches, supplying sensory fibres to a surface area from the vertex of the scalp to the nasolabial junction, including the conjunctiva. The nasociliary nerve is joined by postganglionic fibres from the ciliary ganglion which are derived from the oculomotor nerve.

The *maxillary division* traverses the foramen rotundum, pterygopalatine fossa and infra-orbital canal, emerging on the face. It has meningeal, zygomatic, palatal, alveolar, palpebral, nasal and labial branches. It supplies the skin in the temporal and maxillary regions, upper lip, nasal cavity, hard and soft palate, and also the upper teeth and the vault of the pharynx. Through the pterygopalatine ganglion it receives postganglionic fibres of the facial nerve; some are distributed in the palatine nerves, others enter the zygomatic branch to reach the lacrimal nerve and innervate the lacrimal gland.

The *mandibular division* is a mixed nerve, containing all the trigeminal motor component. It passes through the foramen ovale, gives off a recurrent meningeal branch and the nerve to the medial pterygoid, then divides into anterior and posterior trunks. The anterior trunk provides a sensory buccal nerve, and three motor branches, the masseteric, deep temporal and lateral pterygoid nerves. The posterior trunk divides into auriculotemporal, lingual and inferior alveolar nerves. The mandibular division supplies the lower teeth, the floor of the mouth, the anterior two-thirds of the tongue (ordinary sensation), the skin over the mandible and part of the auricle. The auriculotemporal nerve is joined by postganglionic fibres from the otic ganglion (glosso-

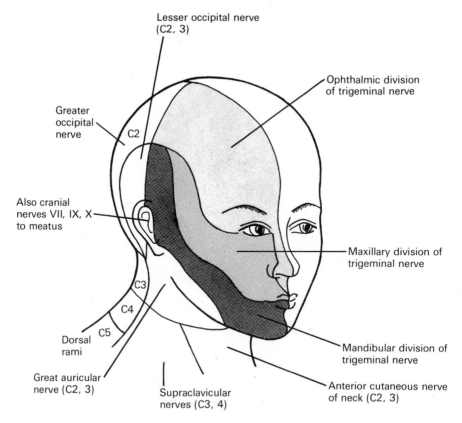

Fig. 6.22 Cutaneous innervation of the head and neck.

pharyngeal) and distributes these to the parotid gland. The lingual nerve is joined by visceral fibres from the chorda tympani (facial nerve). These are afferent and efferent; the afferent component serves taste in the anterior two-thirds of the tongue; the efferent fibres are preganglionic, synapse in the submandibular ganglion and are secretomotor to the submandibular and sublingual glands.

APPLIED ANATOMY

Supranuclear lesions. In connexion with the facial nerve it was noted that hemiplegia may include paralysis of the lower facial muscles. Masticatory muscles would be little affected, since they have bilateral cortical control.

Infranuclear lesions. Peripheral nerve lesions sometimes complicate *skull fractures.* An *aneurysm of the internal carotid artery* in the cavernous sinus may compress the ophthalmic and oculogyric nerves. Occasionally *otitis media* extends to the pneumatic cells in the apex of the petrous temporal bone, affecting the trigeminal ganglion and causing facial pain, and may also involve the abducent nerve, with palsy of the lateral rectus (Gradenigo's syndrome). *Herpes zoster* has a predilection for the trigeminal ophthalmic division in the elderly; two or three days of severe pain are followed by a vesicular (blistered) rash, which starts in the eyebrow and may involve the entire territory of the trigeminal ophthalmic division, but not beyond: thus only half the nose is affected. Herpes frequently causes corneal ulceration; subsequent scarring may produce corneal opacities. *Trigeminal neuralgia* ('tic douloureux') typically occurs in spasmodic attacks of excruciating pain in one or more of the divisions, without sensory loss. Although usually treated medically, an alternative is 'trigeminal tractotomy' which severs connexions with the inferior part of the spinal nucleus mediating pain, but spares touch sensation and, in particular, retains a corneal reflex.

Syringomyelia may cavitate the central canal in the upper cervical cord and lower medulla. The pars caudalis of the trigeminal spinal nucleus may be compressed progressively in a rostral direction, causing the so-called 'onion skin' phenomenon: initially there is analgesia in the posterior part of the face, but this gradually advances anteriorly in concentric zones towards the 'muzzle area', the last to be affected. This process is informative as to spatial representation in the pars caudalis; it does *not* correspond to sequential involvement of trigeminal divisions.

Chapter 7

Cerebellum

GENERAL STRUCTURE

The cerebellum, the largest part of the hindbrain, is in the posterior cranial fossa, beneath the tentorium cerebelli. Centrally it is separated from the pons and medulla by the fourth ventricle. Its surface bears numerous fissures separating narrow *folia* or convolutions, which are mostly transverse. Its appearance is thus very different from that of the cerebral hemispheres. It has two lateral hemispheres, united by a median *vermis (Figs.* 7.1, 7.2, 7.3). The ridge-like *superior vermis* extends anteriorly to the superior medullary velum where it forms the *lingula*. The *inferior vermis* is more clearly demarcated from the hemispheres in the floor of the *vallecula cerebelli*; it is divided by fissures into the *nodule* anteriorly, the *uvula* and part of the *pyramid* posteriorly. From the nodule, on both sides, a stalk extends to the *flocculus* and together these form the *flocculonodular lobe*. The *tonsil* is a partly detached lobule overhanging the inferior

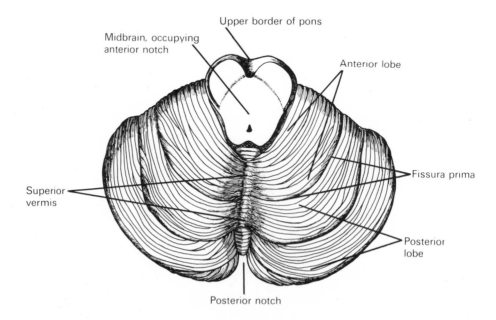

Fig. 7.1 Superior surface of the cerebellum.

132

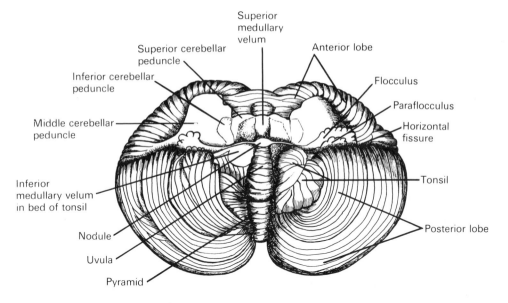

Fig. 7.2 Anteroventral surface of the cerebellum. The right tonsil of the cerebellum has been removed to show the inferior medullary velum.

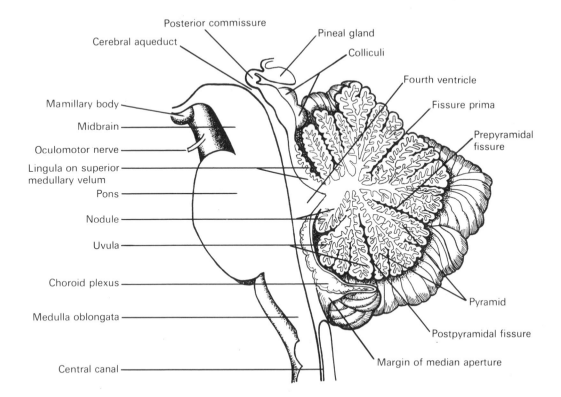

Fig. 7.3 Median sagittal section of the cerebellum and brainstem.

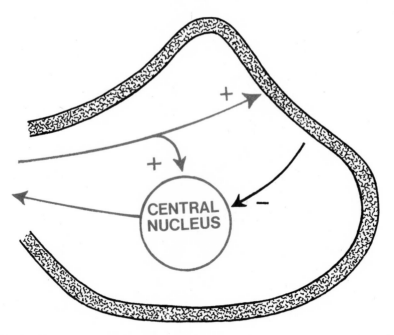

Fig. 7.4 Diagram illustrating excitatory cerebellar input and the inhibitory influence of the cerebellar cortex on the central nuclei.

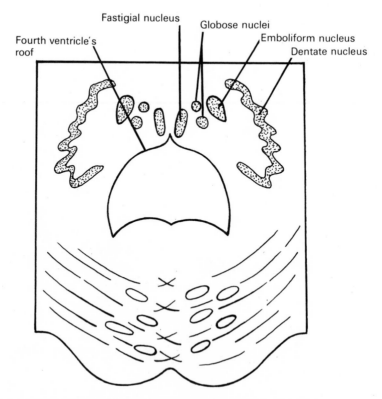

Fig. 7.5 Intracerebellar nuclei in a diagrammatic transverse section.

vermis on each side. Raised intracranial pressure may bulge the tonsils downwards into the foramen magnum.

The cerebellum has three main lobes, *anterior*, *posterior* and *flocculonodular*. On the superior surface a deep V-shaped *fissura prima* is behind the anterior lobe (*Fig.* 7.1). The remainder of the hemispheres, with the pyramid and uvula, forms the posterior lobe. The flocculonodular lobe has been described. A *horizontal fissure* in the posterior lobe demarcates the superior and inferior aspects, and is most evident near the middle cerebellar peduncles and flocculi.

The cerebellum has a grey cortex and a white medullary core in which there are large nuclei. There are three paired peduncles. The superior peduncles ascend into the midbrain, the middle enter from the ventral pons, the inferior ascend from the medulla.

Structurally and functionally the cerebellum reflects evolutionary history. The *archecerebellum* developed with the vestibular nuclei, is concerned with equilibration, is present in fishes, and in man is represented by the flocculonodular lobe and lingula. The *paleocerebellum* emerged with terrestrial vertebrates, which required limbs to support the body against gravity; its input is therefore predominantly spinal and it is linked with locomotion, posture and other stereotyped movements. It includes the anterior lobe and the uvula and pyramids of the posterior lobe. The *neocerebellum* comprises the posterior lobe (except the uvula and pyramids) and is the largest region. It parallels the development of the cerebral hemispheres. Cortico-ponto-cerebellar fibres provide the input for the control of non-stereotyped, skilled and learned activities.

Cerebellar cortical cytoarchitecture is uniform in its details. Afferents project to the cerebellar cortex, whose output is mostly to central nuclei, in which efferent fibres originate (*Fig.* 7.4). The cortex inhibits the nuclei. Afferent fibres provide collaterals to maintain an excitatory state in each intracerebellar nucleus, controlled by varying the inhibition it receives from the cortex; but the vestibular nuclei receive some fibres direct from the cortex.

There are four pairs of nuclei (*Fig.* 7.5) with structural names which long preceded ideas of their functions. The *fastigial nucleus* is near the apex of the roof of the fourth ventricle ('fastigium' is the latin name for the top of a gabled roof). The *globose* (rounded) and *emboliform* (plug-shaped) nuclei are a functional unit. The *dentate nucleus* (toothed in profile) is largest and particularly prominent in man.

Nuclear connexions can be summarized as follows:

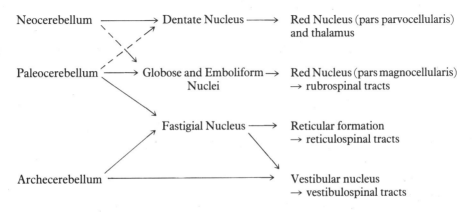

Efferent connexions will be explained later, but note now that the dentate nucleus is particularly associated with the neocerebellum. The globose-emboliform and fastigial nuclei are associated with the paleocerebellum. Primitively the archecerebellum had no central nucleus but some of its efferents relay in the fastigial nucleus. There is some corticonuclear 'exchange' between the three parts of the cerebellum.

THE CEREBELLAR CORTEX

Most of the cortex is submerged between the folia: only about 15% is visible on the surface. The cortex is trilaminar, with molecular, Purkinje (piriform) and granular layers (*Figs. 7.6, 7.7*).

The *molecular layer* is superficial and contains relatively few cells, consisting mainly of fibres: those which run *along* folia are from the granular cells of the deep layer, while those orientated *across* folia are Purkinje cell dendrites. The small cells in the molecular layer are inhibitory interneurons: the *stellate cells* are in the plane of the Purkinje dendrites, and the *basket cells* have a basket-like arborization around the bodies of Purkinje cells.

The *Purkinje (piriform) cells* are very large Golgi Type I neurons whose axons convey cortical output to the central nuclei; they have recurrent collateral branches. From the archecerebellar cortex some axons pass directly to the brainstem vestibular nuclei. The large piriform bodies are *arranged in rows along the folia,* forming a thin layer. Each cell has a much branched dendritic tree, orientated *transverse* to the long axis of its folium; the primary and secondary branches are smooth, but subsequent ones have numerous dendritic spines.

The wide *granular cell layer* consists of great numbers of small neurons whose axons ascend into the molecular layer and, having bifurcated like a T, run longitudinally in the folial axis. Each Purkinje cell's dendritic field contacts thousands of these *parallel fibres*. A few inhibitory interneurons, or *Golgi cells*, are superficial in this layer; their bushy dendritic fields extend into the molecular layer, orientated along and across the folium. Their axons are inhibitory to granular cells.

Cerebellar input fibres are of two types. Firstly, there are *climbing fibres* which convey largely pre-integrated 'information' from the inferior olivary nuclei. Each Purkinje neuron receives only one climbing fibre, but each fibre passes to approximately ten Purkinje neurons – a relatively discrete and non-divergent pattern of input. The inferior olivary nuclei (principal and accessory) receive ascending and descending afferents and project to the whole cerebellar cortex in a series of sagittal strips with a somatotopic organization. *Mossy fibres* are the second type of input fibre and include all other afferents, diverse in origin. The input pattern is highly divergent; thus each fibre divides in a folium to reach both anterior and posterior surfaces, and ends in a bulbous *rosette*, with which the dendrites of many granular cells synapse. Golgi cell axons have an inhibitory effect at this level. The arrangement of the central rosette, granular cell dendrites and Golgi cell axons is a *glomerulus*. Each granular cell axon ascends to the molecular layer, bifurcating there to form fibres parallel to the long axis of the folium.

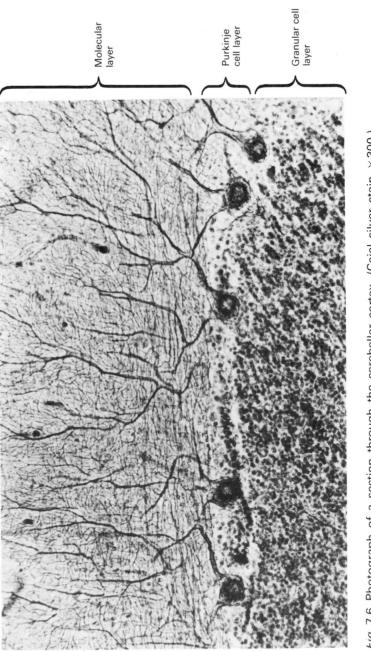

Molecular layer

Purkinje cell layer

Granular cell layer

Fig. 7.6 Photograph of a section through the cerebellar cortex. (Cajal silver stain, ×300.)

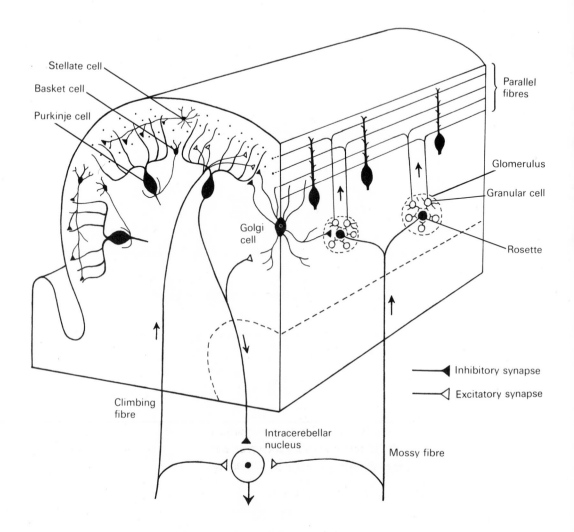

Fig. 7.7 Neuronal organization of the cerebellar cortex.

This complex circuitry is illustrated in *Fig.* 7.8. All afferents are excitatory to the cortex and their collaterals excitatory to the central nuclei. Activity in the mossy fibres creates bands of excitation in the parallel fibres of the molecular layer. When such a band is about as wide as a Purkinje dendritic field, a row of these neurons fire. Synchronously the flanking stellate and basket cells are stimulated and they inhibit adjacent rows of Purkinje cells – a 'neural sharpening' mechanism. The climbing fibres exert more specific influences on individual Purkinje neurons, which transmit a

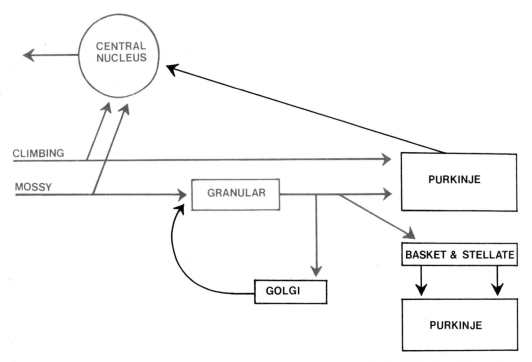

Fig. 7.8 Diagram of neuronal circuitry in the cerebellum: excitation is indicated in red, inhibition in black.

constantly changing pattern of inhibition to the central nuclei. Ascending fibres also activate the Golgi cells, which provide feedback inhibition to the granular cells and thus limit the duration of input. The result is a short discharge from a localized group of Purkinje neurons.

CEREBELLAR PEDUNCLES

Detailed components of the three peduncles are:

Superior peduncle:	Efferent	*Dentato-rubro-thalamic tract* Uncinate fasciculus (aberrant fastigiobulbar)
	Afferent	*Ventral spinocerebellar tract* Tectocerebellar (from inferior colliculus) Trigeminal (mesencephalic nucleus) Rubrocerebellar
Middle peduncle:	Afferent only	*Cortico-ponto-cerebellar* Tectocerebellar (from superior colliculus)
Inferior peduncle:	Afferent	*Inferior olivary nuclei* *Dorsal spinocerebellar tract* Accessory cuneate nucleus Arcuate nuclei Trigeminal
	Afferent and Efferent	*Reticular* *Vestibular*

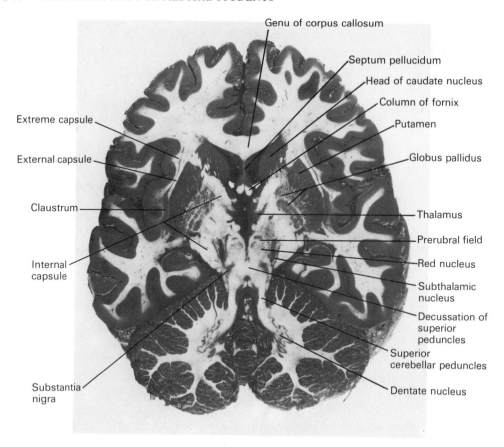

Genu of corpus callosum

Septum pellucidum

Head of caudate nucleus

Column of fornix

Putamen

Globus pallidus

Extreme capsule

External capsule

Claustrum

Internal capsule

Substantia nigra

Thalamus

Prerubral field

Red nucleus

Subthalamic nucleus

Decussation of superior peduncles

Superior cerebellar peduncles

Dentate nucleus

Fig. 7.9 Oblique section through the dentate nuclei and superior cerebellar peduncles. (Mulligan's stain, 0.6 natural size.)

The *superior peduncle*, joining the cerebellum to the midbrain, largely consists of efferent fibres from the dentate nucleus to the contralateral red nucleus and thalamus (*Fig.* 7.9). The *middle peduncle* is the lateral continuation of the transverse fibres of the ventral pons; it is the largest peduncle and contains only afferent fibres. The *inferior peduncle* contains mostly medullary and spinal afferents, but connexions with the vestibular nuclei and reticular formation are reciprocal. This peduncle has two parts, a large lateral *restiform body* and a smaller medial *juxta-restiform body*, the latter consisting of vestibular fibres. As the inferior peduncle ascends from the medulla it turns back between the superior and middle peduncles.

In practice it is essential to recognize that *spinocerebellar connexions are ipsilateral*, and not contralateral as are cerebrospinal connexions.

AFFERENT CONNEXIONS (*Fig.* 7.10)

These may be grouped according to function:

1. *Equilibration.* Vestibulocerebellar fibres are largely from the vestibular nuclei, but some are direct, from the eighth nerve to the archecerebellum

2. *Subconscious proprioception.* Most proprioceptive fibres end in the paleocerebellum, with a topographical localization of the body in the anterior lobe, the feet represented anteriorly, the head posteriorly.

   a. An *ipsilateral* projection from the spinal cord is via *spinocerebellar, cuneocerebellar* and *spino-olivary* paths, and from the face is via the *mesencephalic trigeminal nucleus.* Ventral spinocerebellar fibres which cross in the cord re-cross at cerebellar level to become ipsilateral in the final projection.

   b. *Reticulocerebellar* fibres convey impulses from muscle spindles and from non-specific reticular paths.

   c. *Tectocerebellar* connexions from the superior and inferior colliculi convey visual and auditory impulses concerned with bodily orientation.

3. *Motor control circuits.* The cerebellum co-ordinates muscle groups, smoothes muscle action and adjusts tone by *monitoring* muscular activity. It ensures that the force, direction and extent of movement are appropriate and accurate. It is also involved in the *planning* as well as the control of movement. Motor command signals are relayed through the *cortico-ponto-cerebellar* pathway: most regions of the cerebral cortex project to ipsilateral pontine nuclei via corticopontine tracts; axons from these nuclei

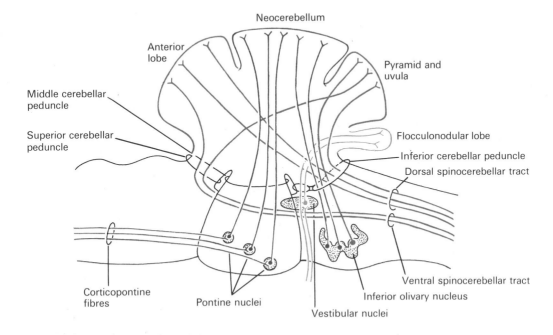

Fig. 7.10 Main afferent cerebellar connexions. Blue: neocerebellum. Red: paleocerebellum. Green: archecerebellum. There are additional afferents, not shown, from the trigeminal nuclei, the tectum and the reticular formation.

cross to form the opposite middle cerebellar peduncle, distributed largely to the neocerebellum. Efferents from the neocerebellar cortex project to the dentate nuclei, from which a *dentato-rubro-thalamic tract* ascends in the superior peduncle (*Fig.* 7.9) to decussate in the midbrain; some fibres end in the contralateral red nucleus, but most reach the thalamus (ventral lateral nucleus) and relay to the motor cortex, modulating activity in the pyramidal and extrapyramidal tracts.

The inferior olivary nuclei receive descending fibres from the cerebral cortex, red nuclei and other brainstem centres. *Olivocerebellar* fibres cross to enter the contralateral inferior peduncle.

EFFERENT CONNEXIONS (*Fig.* 7.11)

1. *Cerebral cortex*. The dentato-rubro-thalamic route to the cortex has been described.
2. *Red nucleus*. The red nucleus has a caudal part containing large and small cells (pars magnocellularis) and a phylogenetically more recent rostral region of small cells (pars parvocellularis). The neocerebellum and dentate nucleus project to the pars parvocellularis; the paleocerebellum projects through the globose and emboliform nuclei to the pars magnocellularis, in which descending fibres arise. *Rubrospinal* and *rubrobulbar* tracts cross in the midbrain as the *ventral tegmental decussation*; *rubroreticular* fibres contribute to the reticulospinal tracts.

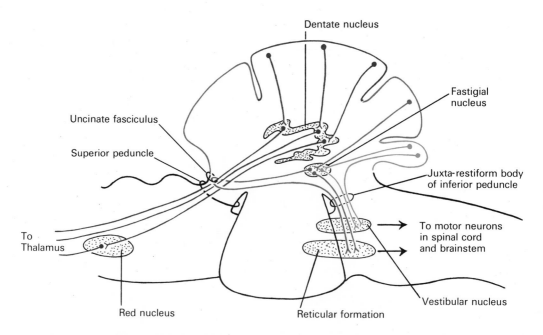

Fig. 7.11 Main efferent cerebellar connexions. Blue: neocerebellum. Red: paleo-cerebellum. Green: archecerebellum. Rubrospinal connexions are not shown.

3. *Reticular formation*. The main outflow from the paleocerebellum and fastigial nucleus to the reticular formation is via the inferior peduncle. Aberrant fastigiobulbar fibres form the *uncinate fasciculus* which hooks over the superior peduncle en route to the reticular formation and vestibular nuclei. Reticulospinal tracts influence muscle tone by the γ control system.
4. *Vestibular nuclei*. Some efferents from the archecerebellum project directly to the vestibular nuclei, others via the fastigial nucleus. Equilibratory control is effected via the vestibulospinal tracts and the medial longitudinal fasciculus.

APPLIED ANATOMY

Cerebellar dysfunction may be due to vascular occlusion, neoplastic invasion or demyelinating disease. The clinical signs are ipsilateral if the lesion is unilateral. The symptoms are most obvious when onset is sudden.

Ataxia (inco-ordination of movement) appears in several forms. In reaching for an object there is *intention tremor* and *dysmetria* shown by 'overshoot' (past-pointing) or 'undershoot'. *Decomposition* of movements into a series of irregular jerky actions appears with an inability to make rapidly alternating movements such as pronation-supination. *Scanning speech* is jerky, slow and slurred, its sounds too loud or too soft, too long or too short. *Nystagmus* is an ataxia of the ocular muscles, inability to fixate resulting in lateral tremor of the eyes. Disturbed equilibrium results in *staggering gait* and a tendency to fall. *Hypotonia* (reduced tone) of muscles is accompanied by weak tendon reflexes.

There are two main sites of lesion, the median vermis and the cerebellar hemispheres. A *vermal lesion* leads to disequilibrium and nystagmus. In children a rapidly growing tumour (medulloblastoma) may affect the vermis, resulting in ataxia of the trunk so severe that the child cannot sit up or hold up its head. Disease of one *cerebellar hemisphere* results in ipsilateral ataxia and hypotonia, becoming more severe, with intention tremor, if either the dentate nucleus or the superior peduncle are involved.

Chapter 8

Diencephalon and internal capsule

The diencephalon comprises the thalamus, hypothalamus, subthalamus and epithalamus. On each side it extends anteroposteriorly from the interventricular foramen to the posterior commissure, and transversely from the internal capsule to the ependymal lining of the third ventricle.

THALAMUS

The thalami form the largest part of the diencephalon. Each is narrow and rounded anteriorly, where it lies just behind the interventricular foramen. Its expanded posterior end is named the *pulvinar*, and overhangs the superior colliculus. The medial surface adjoins the third ventricle; a shallow *hypothalamic sulcus* between the interventricular foramen and aqueduct is a boundary between the thalamus and hypothalamus (*Fig.* 8.1). The subthalamus is between the thalamus and midbrain. The thalami are usually attached across the midline by a narrow *interthalamic connexus* of grey matter. The superior surface is grooved by the fornix, lateral to which the thalamus forms part of the lateral ventricle's floor (*Fig.* 8.10). The junction of the superior and medial surfaces is marked by a band of white fibres, the *stria medullaris thalami*.

Thalamic nuclei (*Figs.* 8.2, 8.3)

Thalamic grey matter is partially divided into medial and lateral regions by an oblique white sheet, the *internal medullary lamina*. Anteriorly this splits to enclose an *anterior nucleus*. The medial region has a large *dorsal medial nucleus* and a small group of *median nuclei*. The lateral part is divided into dorsal and ventral tiers of nuclei; the dorsal tier is subdivided craniocaudally into the *lateral dorsal* and *lateral posterior nuclei* and a large caudal nuclear mass which forms the *pulvinar*; the ventral tier is subdivided into *ventral anterior (VA)*, *ventral lateral (VL)* and *ventral posterior (VP) nuclei*. There are also central *intralaminar nuclei*, the largest being the *centromedian nucleus*. The *reticular nucleus* is a thin curved sheet on the lateral aspect of the thalamus, separated from it by white fibres of the *external medullary lamina*. The medial and lateral *geniculate nuclei*, forming the *metathalamus*, are posteroventral to the pulvinar.

The thalamic nuclei may be placed in three main functional groups: specific, non-specific and reticular.

144

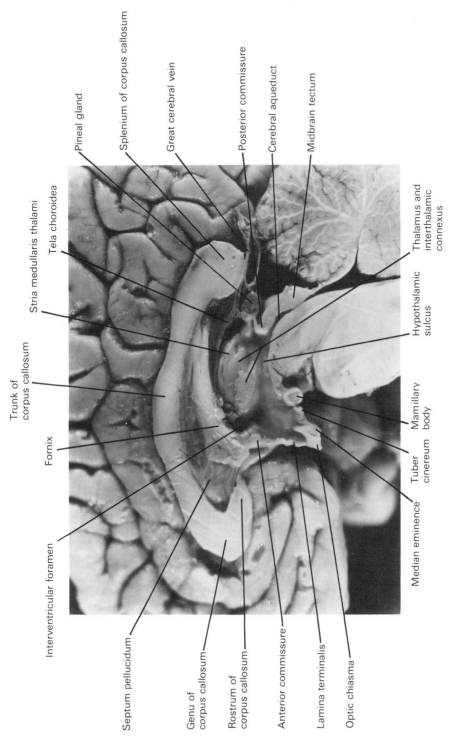

Stria medullaris thalami

Tela choroidea

Pineal gland

Splenium of corpus callosum

Great cerebral vein

Posterior commissure

Cerebral aqueduct

Midbrain tectum

Trunk of corpus callosum

Interventricular foramen

Fornix

Thalamus and interthalamic connexus

Hypothalamic sulcus

Septum pellucidum

Genu of corpus callosum

Rostrum of corpus callosum

Anterior commissure

Lamina terminalis

Optic chiasma

Median eminence

Tuber cinereum

Mamillary body

Fig. 8.1 Median sagittal section of the brain illustrating the relationships of the diencephalon (×1.05).

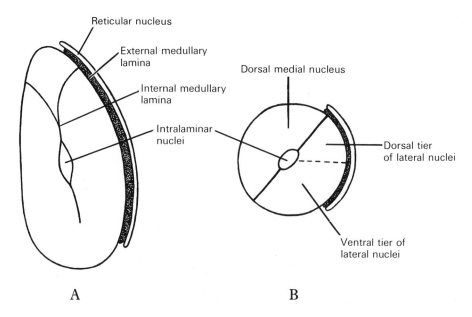

Fig. 8.2 Diagrams of the right thalamus in horizontal section (A) and
in coronal section (B).

Specific nuclei

These receive specific forms of input from certain ascending tracts and project to
specific ('primary') cortical areas. They degenerate after ablation of those areas. They
are both sensory (VP and geniculate) and motor (VA, VL).

1. *Ventral Posterior Nucleus (VP).* This receives ascending somatic sensory fibres. Its
   lateral division receives the medial lemniscus and spinothalamic tracts, its medial
   division trigeminothalamic fibres and secondary gustatory fibres from the nucleus
   solitarius. Thus the head is represented medially, the feet laterally. These nuclei
   project to the postcentral gyrus in which the body is inverted. There are also
   connexions to the dorsal tier nuclei (integration) and the dorsal medial nucleus
   (emotional response).
2. *Geniculate Nuclei.* The medial geniculate nucleus receives auditory fibres from the
   inferior colliculus via the inferior brachium, projecting via the auditory radiation to
   the primary auditory cortex in the floor of the lateral fissure and the superior
   temporal gyrus.

   The lateral geniculate nucleus receives most fibres of the optic tract, projecting via
   the optic radiation to the primary visual cortex in the occipital lobe. It has a complex
   six-layered structure and will be considered with the visual system.
3. *Ventral Lateral (VL) and Ventral Anterior (VA) Nuclei.* These are both concerned with
   motor control, receiving afferents from the cerebellum (via the dentato-rubro-
   thalamic tract), the corpus striatum and the substantia nigra. They project to the
   motor cortex (precentral gyrus and premotor area) and contribute to the initiation

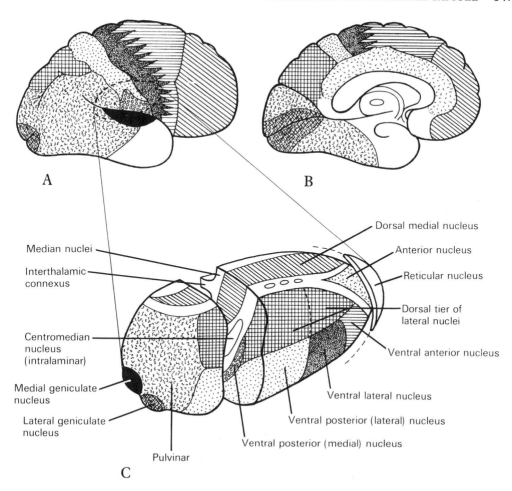

A

B

Dorsal medial nucleus

Median nuclei

Anterior nucleus

Interthalamic connexus

Reticular nucleus

Dorsal tier of lateral nuclei

Centromedian nucleus (intralaminar)

Ventral anterior nucleus

Medial geniculate nucleus

Ventral lateral nucleus

Lateral geniculate nucleus

Ventral posterior (lateral) nucleus

Ventral posterior (medial) nucleus

Pulvinar

C

Fig. 8.3 Cortical projections of the thalamic nuclei. (A) Right lateral view of the cerebrum. (B) Median sagittal aspect of the same. (C) Dorsolateral view of the right thalamus showing the arrangement of the nuclei. Equivalent shading patterns indicate the relationships between thalamic nuclei and the cortical areas they influence. (After Warwick R. and Williams P. L. (1973) *Gray's Anatomy*, 35th ed. Edinburgh, Longman.)

and control of movement. Parkinson's disease is associated with degenerative change in the substantia nigra: the resultant tremor and rigidity can be reduced surgically by an electrolytic lesion placed in the VL nucleus.

Non-specific nuclei

These do not receive ascending tracts, but have abundant connexions with other diencephalic nuclei, projecting mostly to cortical 'association areas' in the frontal and parietal lobes and, to a lesser extent, in the occipital and temporal lobes. The cortical association areas are concerned with the correlation and interpretation of information.

1. *Dorsal Medial Nucleus*. This, the largest sub-nucleus in the medial thalamic region, is highly developed in primates and especially in man. It receives afferents from other thalamic nuclei and from the hypothalamus. It integrates somatic and visceral afferents and has reciprocal connexions with the prefrontal cortex (frontal association area). It is associated with mood and emotional balance; depending on the nature of current sensory input and previous experience, feelings of euphoria or depression may result. Through its hypothalamic connexions, visceral response to emotion may occur: an unpleasant sight may cause vomiting; tension and apprehension may lead to anorexia or diarrhoea. In psychosomatic disorders, patients appear with apparently physical illnesses of psychogenic origin. Serious depressive illness has, in the past, been relieved by prefrontal leucotomy, by which the connexions between the dorsal medial nucleus and the prefrontal cortex are severed. The operation has undesirable side effects and is now largely replaced by anti-depressive drugs.

    Memory defects may follow damage to this thalamic region.
2. *Anterior Nucleus*. This receives afferents from the hypothalamus via the *mamillo-thalamic tract*, and projects through the anterior limb of the internal capsule to the *cingulate gyrus*. It is part of the limbic system, described later, which is concerned with the emotional drives and instinctive behaviour necessary to preservation of the individual and the species. It also has an essential role in memory activity.
3. *Dorsal Tier of Lateral Nuclei*. These receive input from the ventral tier and have reciprocal connexions with the association areas in the parietal, occipital and temporal lobes. They are involved in the analysis and integration of sensory input. Visual and auditory information are correlated in the pulvinar.

Nuclei connected with the reticular formation

1. *Reticular Nucleus*. This thin lateral thalamic sheet of cells is a rostral extension of the brainstem reticular formation. It has diffuse reciprocal connexions with the whole cerebral cortex and other thalamic nuclei, being part of the *reticular activating system*.
2. *Intralaminar Nuclei*. The internal medullary lamina encloses several nuclei, the largest being the *centromedian nucleus* (*Fig. 8.3, 8.9*). These receive reticular afferents via the central tegmental tract and project to other thalamic nuclei and to the corpus striatum. Stimulation evokes an 'arousal response', shown by encephalography. These nuclei profoundly affect the level of consciousness and alertness. They are also involved in the awareness of painful stimuli at thalamic level; intractable pain may be relieved by electrolytic destruction of them, although this also results in somnolence.
3. *Median Nuclei*. This is a relatively small group in man. They are in the wall of the third ventricle above the hypothalamic sulcus and in the thalamic connexus. They receive visceral afferents from the reticular formation, and are connected with the hypothalamus (visceral response), dorsal medial nucleus (emotional reaction) and intralaminar nuclei (arousal).

Summary of thalamic functions

Most of the cerebral cortex is influenced by the thalamus and most thalamic nuclei receive impulses from the cortex.

1. *Sensory integration and relay.* All forms of sensory input (except olfactory) converge on the thalamus, where they are correlated into an integrated pattern projected to the cortex.
2. *Motor integration and relay.* The corpus striatum, substantia nigra and cerebellum exert their influence on the corticospinal and corticobulbar motor pathways via the thalamus.
3. *Awareness of nociceptive stimuli* occurs in non-discriminative form at thalamic level. In thalamic lesions, or if cortical influence is removed, the peripheral pain threshold is raised and the response is excessive. Spontaneous pain is sometimes a feature of thalamic disorders.
4. *Emotional and subjective responses* to sensation. Somatic input is interpreted as agreeable or disagreeable. Connexions with the frontal cortex are important in determining mood.
5. *Memory and instinctive behaviour.* The anterior nucleus is part of the limbic system.
6. *Activation and arousal.* Thalamic reticular components generate much of the low voltage, rapid, desynchronized cortical activity seen in the encephalograms of alert individuals.

APPLIED ANATOMY

Functional and applied aspects of individual thalamic nuclei have already been described. Vascular occlusion results in a *thalamic syndrome* of combined sensory and emotional symptoms, their severity depending on the extent of the lesion. Sensation from the contralateral side of the body is impaired, its threshold raised, and when perceived it is exaggerated and unpleasant. This may be accompanied by marked emotional instability. Failing blood supply may precipitate spontaneous and intractable pain in the opposite side of the body; surgical destruction of the ventral posterior nucleus relieves this but results in hemianaesthesia and, if the cerebellar projection to the ventral lateral nucleus is damaged, in atonia and ataxia.

Thalamic radiations and the internal capsule (*Figs.* 8.4, 8.5, 9.2)

In horizontal section, the internal capsule is a compact aggregation of fibres sited between the thalamus and caudate nucleus medially and the lentiform nucleus laterally. It has an anterior limb, genu and posterior limb and retrolentiform and sublentiform parts. It consists of motor and sensory cortical projection fibres. Between the internal capsule and the cortex these fibres diverge as the *corona radiata*.

Fibres reciprocally connecting the thalamus and cortex are the *thalamic radiations*. The *anterior radiation*, in the anterior limb of the internal capsule, connects the anterior and dorsal medial thalamic nuclei with frontal cortex. The *superior radiation* is in the posterior limb and connects the ventral tier nuclei with the primary sensory cortex (VP nucleus) and with the precentral gyrus and premotor cortex (VL, VA nuclei). The *posterior radiation* occupies the retrolentiform part of the internal capsule, projecting from the lateral geniculate nucleus to the primary visual cortex of the occipital lobe as the optic radiation. It also includes many fibres between the pulvinar and the visual

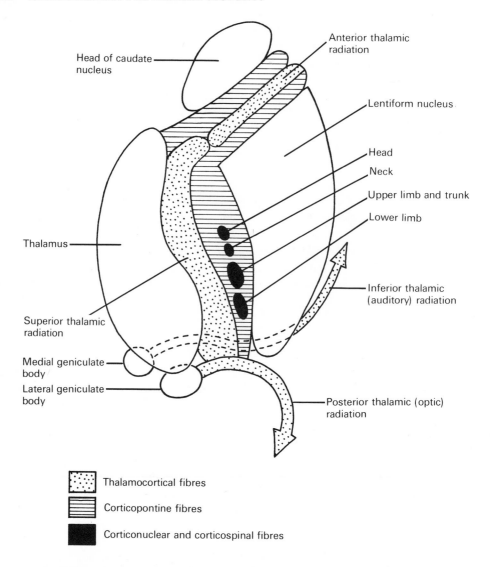

Fig. 8.4 Diagram of the components of the right internal capsule. (After Carpenter M. B. and Sutin J. (1981) *Human Neuroanatomy*. Baltimore, Williams and Wilkins.)

association cortex. The *inferior radiation* is the sublentiform part of the internal capsule, mostly formed by the auditory radiation, from the medial geniculate nucleus to the temporal auditory cortex. It also contains connexions between the pulvinar and the auditory association cortex.

Corticofugal fibres descending in the internal capsule are corticopontine, pyramidal (corticospinal, corticonuclear), and extrapyramidal.

Corticopontine fibres have widespread origins in the cerebral cortex. Frontopontine fibres occupy the anterior and posterior limbs of the internal capsule, temporopontine and parietopontine fibres its posterior limb and sublentiform part. These fibres synapse

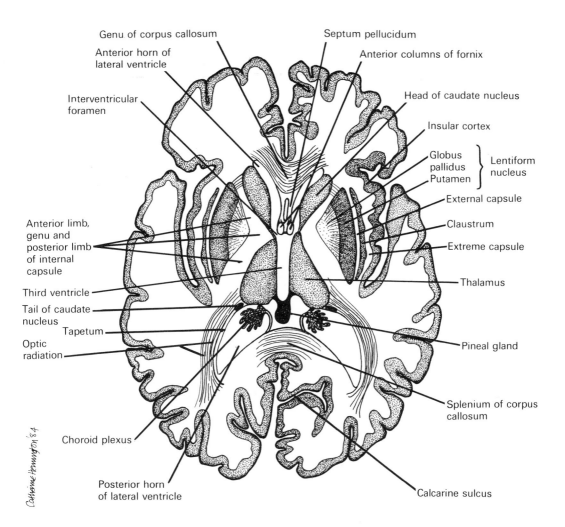

Fig. 8.5 Horizontal section of the cerebrum at the level of the interventricular foramen. (Compare with a photographed section, *Fig.* 9.2.)

with the ipsilateral pontine nuclei, from which axons cross to the contralateral cerebellar hemisphere in its middle peduncle.

Corticonuclear fibres (to cranial motor nuclei) are just behind the genu in the internal capsule; *corticospinal* fibres are in the posterior half of its posterior limb.

Extrapyramidal fibres are named according to their destinations; there are cortico-striate, corticorubral, cortico-olivary, corticonigral and corticoreticular fibres. Most appear to lie near the corticospinal tracts and are affected in lesions of the posterior limb of the internal capsule. However, some corticostriate and corticoreticular fibres are in the external capsule.

APPLIED ANATOMY

The internal capsule receives blood largely from the striate branches of the middle cerebral artery and the anterior choroidal artery. Thrombosis or haemorrhage of them results in widespread neurological dysfunction. A lesion in the posterior limb of the internal capsule causes contralateral upper motor lesion effects (hemiplegia), sometimes with partial sensory loss. A vascular lesion in the retrolentiform region produces blindness in the contralateral visual field.

SUBTHALAMUS (*Figs.* 8.6, 8.7, 8.8, 8.9)

The subthalamic region, a transitional zone between the midbrain and the diencephalon, lies posterior to the hypothalamus, adjoining the thalamus and internal capsule. Ascending tracts such as the medial lemniscus traverse it en route to the thalamus. The red nucleus extends into it, and the dentato-rubro-thalamic tract is part of the *thalamic fasciculus* in the prerubral field, between the red nucleus and the thalamus.

The *subthalamic nucleus*, which looks like a biconvex lens in coronal section, is closely related to the medial aspect of the internal capsule, which separates it from the globus pallidus of corpus striatum. The subthalamic nucleus and globus pallidus are inter-connected by the *subthalamic fasciculus*, which traverses the internal capsule.

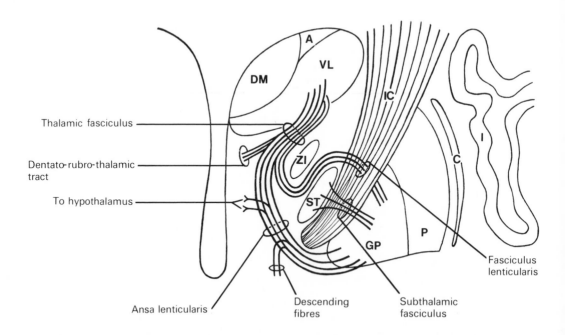

Fig. 8.6 Fibre tracts in the subthalamus. **VL**, Ventral lateral thalamic nucleus; **A**, Anterior thalamic nucleus; **DM**, Dorsal medial thalamic nucleus; **IC**, Internal capsule; **ZI**, Zona incerta; **ST**, Subthalamic nucleus; **GP**, Globus pallidus; **P**, Putamen; **C**, Claustrum; **I**, Insula.

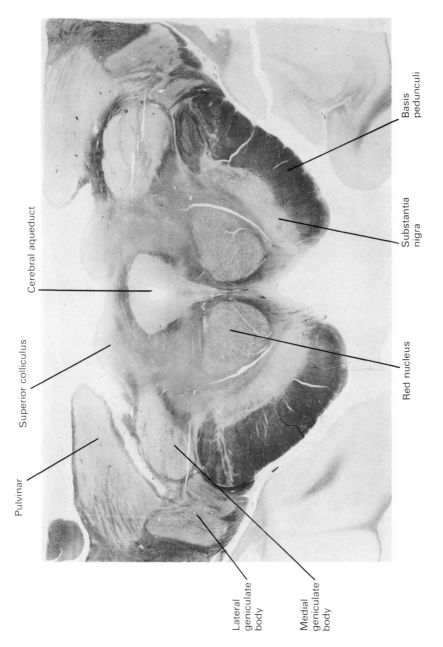

Fig. 8.7 Transverse section through the upper midbrain. (Weigert stain, × 3.)

Basis pedunculi

Substantia nigra

Red nucleus

Cerebral aqueduct

Superior colliculus

Pulvinar

Lateral geniculate body

Medial geniculate body

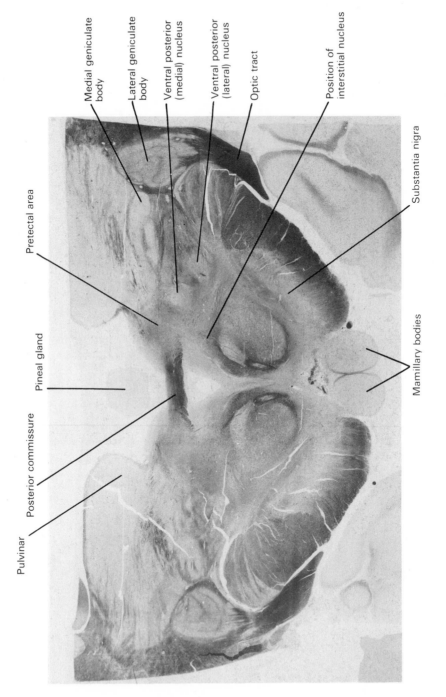

Fig. 8.8 Transverse section at the junction of the mesencephalon and diencephalon. (Weigert stain, ×3.)

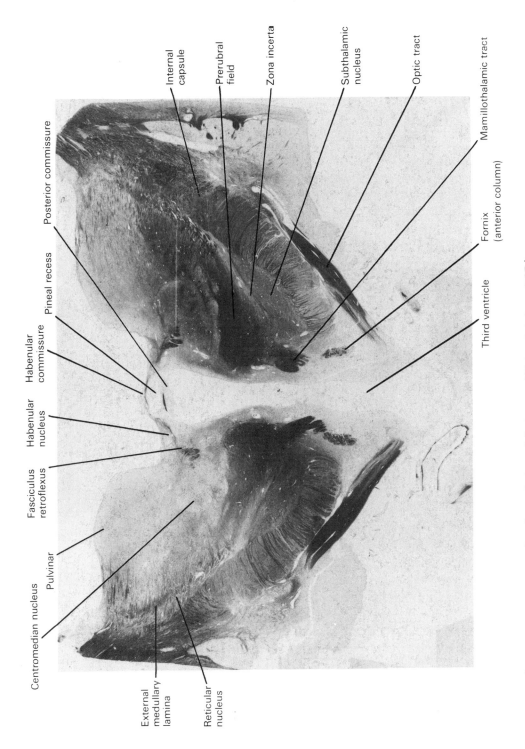

Fig. 8.9 Oblique transverse section through the subthalamus. (Weigert stain, × 2.25.)

The *zona incerta* is a rostral extension of the midbrain reticular formation and a continuation of the thalamic reticular nucleus. It is between the thalamus and the subthalamic nucleus, partly surrounded by tracts of nerve fibres (*Fig.* 8.6).

The globus pallidus is the efferent part of the corpus striatum; fibres connecting it to the thalamus traverse this region in two fasciculi. The *fasciculus lenticularis* pierces the internal capsule and arches round the zona incerta to join the thalamic fasciculus; the *ansa lenticularis* curves medially round the ventral border of the internal capsule to enter the prerubral field and reach the thalamus. Descending fibres pass from the ansa lenticularis to the substantia nigra and the midbrain reticular formation.

APPLIED ANATOMY

The subthalamic nucleus is an important extrapyramidal component; it exerts an inhibitory effect on the globus pallidus. Damage to this nucleus, although rare, has dramatic effects. Unilateral, it induces wild flinging movements (*hemiballismus*) in the contralateral limbs, particularly affecting the shoulder joint, so violent that one patient broke her arm against the side of the cot (Patten, 1977). It may be relieved either medically or by stereotactic surgery to the fasciculus lenticularis or globus pallidus.

EPITHALAMUS

The epithalamus includes structures lying posteriorly in the diencephalic roof such as the *habenular nuclei, posterior commissure* and *pineal gland* (Fig. 8.10).

Each *habenular nucleus* occupies the floor of its *habenular trigone*. Afferents reach it in the *stria medullaris thalami*, fibres applied to the dorsomedial thalamic surface (*Fig.* 8.1). These afferents, of diverse origin, are associated with the olfactory or limbic systems, including connexions with the septal area and amygdaloid nucleus (via the stria terminalis) and from the hippocampal formation (via the fornix). These structures are described in Chapter 10. Some fibres of the stria medullaris cross in the *habenular commissure* and interconnect the hippocampal or the amygdaloid centres. Habenular efferents form the *fasciculus retroflexus*, which ends in the midbrain interpeduncular nucleus. This projects to the tegmental nuclei and via the *dorsal longitudinal fasciculus* to the autonomic centres of the brainstem controlling salivation, gastrointestinal motility and secretion, a pathway by which olfaction and emotion effect visceral responses.

The *posterior commissure* (*Figs.* 8.1, 8.8, 8.11), just below the pineal stalk, is a composite connexion between the medial longitudinal fasciculi, interstitial nuclei, superior colliculi, pretectal nuclei and posterior thalamic nuclei.

The *pineal gland* is a midline structure overhanging the superior colliculi and below the splenium of the corpus callosum, from which it is separated by the great cerebral vein (*Fig.* 8.1). It is attached to the diencephalon by a *stalk*, invaded by a *pineal recess* of the third ventricle; its lower part is attached to the posterior commissure, the upper part contains the habenular commissure. Pinealocytes and neuroglial cells form the gland. Sympathetic fibres from the superior cervical ganglion influence pinealocyte secretion

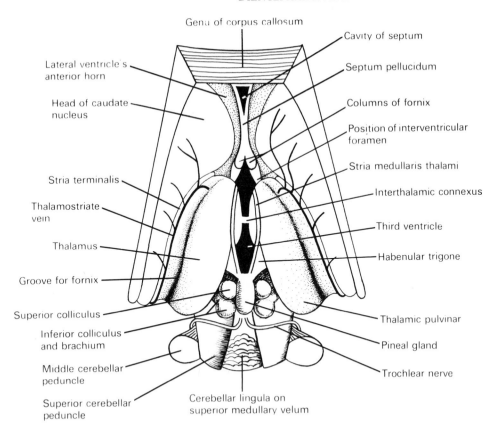

Fig. 8.10 The thalami, caudate nuclei and third ventricle, seen from above after removal of most of the corpus callosum, the body of the fornix and the tela choroidea.

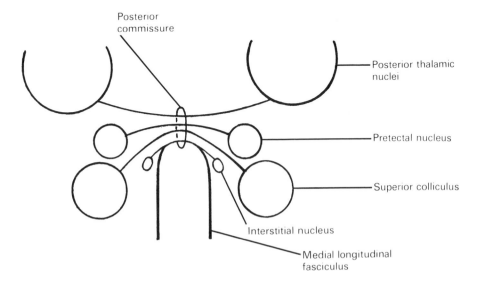

Fig. 8.11 Diagram of the composition of the posterior commissure.

of *melatonin* and *serotonin*, which may enter cerebrospinal fluid or capillaries. In some fishes, amphibians and reptiles, the pineal gland is subcutaneous and contains photoreceptors. Melatonin affects the melanocytes, altering the skin colour in these creatures. Diurnal fluctuation of pineal secretion occurs in mammals, but the effect of light is by an indirect route: the hypothalamus receives retinal afferents and influences sympathetic neurons via the superior cervical ganglion. Melatonin does not affect human skin colour.

APPLIED ANATOMY

Pineal secretion is *anti-gonadotrophic*: pineal destruction in immature individuals leads to precocious puberty; conversely, a secreting pineal tumour delays its onset. Whether pineal hormones exert this effect via the hypothalamus or the adenohypophysis is unknown. An expanding pineal tumour may compress the pretectal region and superior colliculi, producing fixed, dilated pupils and loss of upward gaze. In the adult, calcareous aggregations accumulate in the gland (a useful midline marker in radiograms).

HYPOTHALAMUS

Basic structure

The hypothalamus occupies the basal diencephalic region forming the lower part of the lateral wall and floor of the third ventricle (*Fig.* 8.1). The hypothalamic sulcus, between the interventricular foramen and the aqueduct, marks its dorsal boundary. It extends posteriorly from the lamina terminalis to the midbrain tegmentum. Posterolaterally is the subthalamus. The ventral region between the optic chiasma and the *mamillary bodies* is the *tuber cinereum*. The pituitary gland is attached by a stalk (infundibulum) to a *median eminence* immediately behind the optic chiasma. The hypothalamus consists of (bilateral) medial and lateral zones: between them an anterior column of the fornix arches down to each mamillary body.

Lateral zone (*Fig.* 8.12B)

This is traversed by the longitudinal fibres of the *medial forebrain bundle* which interconnects the septal area and hypothalamus and projects to reticular nuclei in the midbrain tegmentum. It contains an extensive *lateral nucleus* and smaller *supra-optic*, *tuberomamillary* and *lateral tuberal* nuclei, and has more fibres and fewer neurons than the medial zone.

Medial zone (*Fig.* 8.12A)

This contains many neurons, in nuclei, gathered into anterior, tuberal and posterior groups, the anterior including the *pre-optic*, *supra-optic*, *paraventricular* and *anterior*

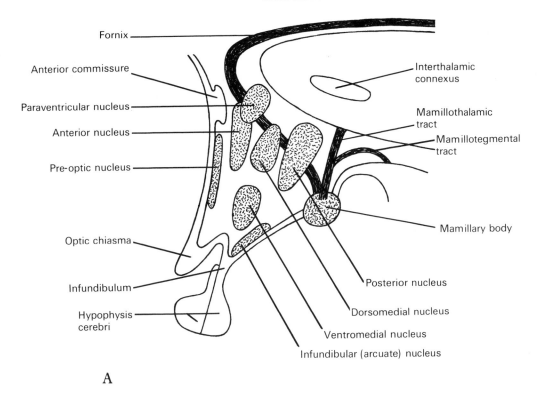

Fornix

Anterior commissure

Paraventricular nucleus

Anterior nucleus

Pre-optic nucleus

Optic chiasma

Infundibulum

Hypophysis
cerebri

Interthalamic
connexus

Mamillothalamic
tract

Mamillotegmental
tract

Mamillary body

Posterior nucleus

Dorsomedial nucleus

Ventromedial nucleus

Infundibular (arcuate) nucleus

A

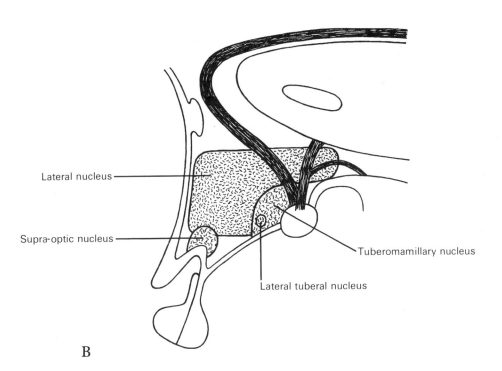

Lateral nucleus

Supra-optic nucleus

Tuberomamillary nucleus

Lateral tuberal nucleus

B

Fig. 8.12 Hypothalamic nuclei. (A) Medial zone. (B) Lateral zone.

nuclei. Axons of neurons in the supra-optic and paraventricular nuclei extend to the neurohypophysis as a *supraoptico-hypophysial tract*; hormone precursors, formed within the cells of the nuclei, are transported along this tract to the neurohypophysis. This anterior region also exerts control over the parasympathetic system. The tuberal region includes *dorsomedial*, *ventromedial* and *infundibular* nuclei, and has diffuse metabolic functions; it has a 'centre' responding to hunger and a 'satiety centre'. The *tubero-hypophysial tract* carries 'releasing factors' to the median eminence, transported thence to the adenohypophysis in a *portal system*, each factor effecting release (or inhibition) of a particular hormone. The posterior group includes the *mamillary nuclei* and *posterior nucleus*; a sympathetic control 'centre' is located posteriorly in the hypothalamus.

Afferent connexions

1. *Visceral and somatic afferents.* General visceral afferents arrive from the vagal sensory nucleus, gustatory afferents from the nucleus solitarius, and somatic afferents from the nipples and genitalia. Retinal afferents, concerned with light intensity, programme a 'biological clock'.
2. *Olfactory input* is mostly via the medial forebrain bundle.
3. *Limbic system, thalamus and cortex.* The hippocampus, in the floor of the inferior horn of the lateral ventricle is connected by the *fornix* to the mamillary body, with collaterals to other hypothalamic nuclei. The amygdaloid nucleus, in the roof of the inferior horn, has efferents forming the *stria terminalis* which reach the anterior hypothalamic and septal regions. Both these tracts, the fornix and the stria curve round the thalamus (*Figs. 8.1, 8.10, 10.2*). The *medial forebrain bundle* brings afferents from the septal region. The *mamillothalamic tract* connects the hypo-thalamus to the anterior thalamic nucleus, which projects to the cingulate gyrus. These are all part of the limbic system, forming a border (limbus), around the junction of the diencephalon and prosencephalon.

    The dorsal medial thalamic nucleus and prefrontal cortex transmit emotional, affective information to the hypothalamus via a periventricular system of fibres on the medial surface of the thalamus.
4. *Direct physical and chemical receptors.* Circulating blood is constantly monitored by hypothalamic cells, which function as thermoreceptors, osmoreceptors or chemoreceptors.

Efferent connexions

The hypothalamus influences three main regions: autonomic, thalamic-limbic and hypophysial (pituitary).
1. *Autonomic control.* The *mamillotegmental tract* arches caudally from the mamillary body to the midbrain tegmentum (*Fig. 8.12*); some efferent fibres also reach the tegmentum in the medial forebrain bundle and periventricular fibres, entering the *dorsal longitudinal fasciculus* and reticular nuclei. Tegmental efferents pass to parasympathetic nuclei in the brainstem (salivatory, lacrimal and dorsal vagal motor nuclei) and to spinal autonomic nuclei. These visceral pathways were considered,

until recently, to be entirely polysynaptic, but some axons extend from the hypothalamus to the medulla and spinal cord.

2. *Thalamus and Limbic System.* The mamillothalamic tract projects to the anterior thalamic nucleus and is thence connected to the cingulate gyrus, as part of the limbic system, whose function may be summarized as the preservation of the individual and the species. Other connexions between the hypothalamus and the limbic system, already described, contain both afferent and efferent fibres. Connexions between the hypothalamus, the dorsal medial thalamic nucleus and the prefrontal cortex are also reciprocal.

3. *Hypophysis Cerebri*
   a. *Neurohypophysis.* The supra-optic and paraventricular nuclei project to the posterior lobe of the hypophysis as the supraoptico-hypophysial tract (*Fig. 8.13A*); their cells secrete precursors of oxytocin and vasopressin, transported as granules (Herring bodies) by axoplasmic flow along the tract for release into the capillaries of the neurohypophysis. *Oxytocin* causes contraction of uterine muscle and mammary myo-epithelial cells, effects demonstrable after parturition when a baby is put to the breast. *Vasopressin (antidiuretic hormone)*, a vasoconstrictor, has an important antidiuretic effect on the renal distal convoluted tubules. Osmoreceptors and a 'thirst centre' are near the supra-optic nucleus; destruction here results in diabetes insipidus, in which the volume of urine is excessive. Individual nuclei were considered specialized for the production of a single hormone, but it is now known that both hormones are produced in each nucleus.
   b. *Adenohypophysis.* The *tubero-infundibular tract* (*Fig. 8.13B*) ends in the median eminence and infundibulum. 'Releasing factors', formed in the tuberal and infundibular nuclei, are carried to the adenohypophysis in a *hypophysial portal system* formed from hypophysial branches of the internal carotid artery entering the median eminence to divide into tufts of capillaries; from these, blood traverses the portal veins to a plexus of sinusoidal capillaries among the cells of the adenohypophysis. The releasing factors are each specific to corticotrophin, luteinizing hormone, follicular stimulating hormone, thyrotrophin and somato-trophin. They may promote synthesis as well as release; they inhibit the release of prolactin and melanocyte stimulating hormone.

Summary of hypothalamic functions

1. *Autonomic control.* Stimulation of the sympathetic or parasympathetic hypothalmic 'centres' affects the cardiovascular, respiratory and alimentary systems. The anterior hypothalamus responds to hyperthermia by causing vasodilatation, sweating and lowered metabolism, while its posterior region responds to hypothermia by causing vasoconstriction, shivering and increased thyroid activity. This thermostatic control is less efficient in the very young and the very old. Circulating bacterial pyrogens stimulate hypothalamic chemoreceptors to produce the febrile response.

2. *Endocrine control.* The hypothalamic centres are sensitive to circulatory hormonal levels, providing negative or positive feedbacks. Neural paths converging on the

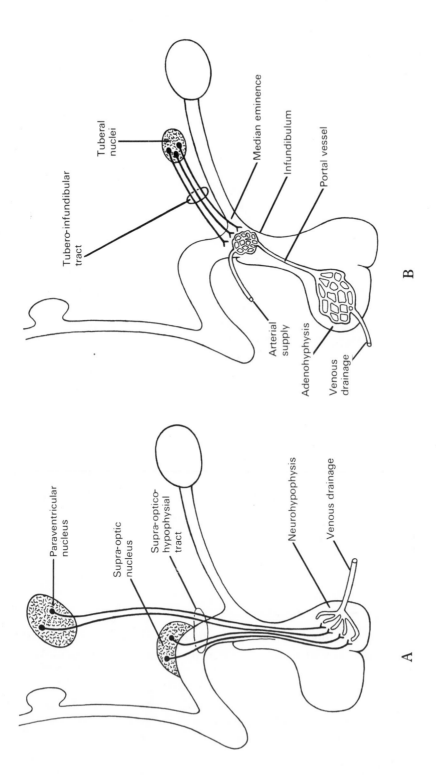

Fig. 8.13 Hypothalamo-hypophysial control mechanisms.
(A) Supraoptico-hypophysial tract to neurohypophysis. (B) Hypophysial portal system to adenohypophysis.

hypothalamus also influence hormonal release. Some hypophysial hormones directly affect their target tissues, others, such as ACTH, act through an endocrine intermediary.

3. *Food and water intake.* Stimulation of the lateral hypothalamus promotes eating; ablation may lead to death from starvation. Conversely, stimulation of the medial tuberal region causes anorexia. Thus a lateral '*hunger centre*' is functionally balanced against a medial '*satiety centre*'. A '*thirst centre*' in the lateral region regulates fluid intake, influencing renal secretion by regulating the production of antidiuretic hormone.

4. *Emotional expression.* The hypothalamus, informed by the limbic system, prefrontal cortex and other central nervous regions mediates autonomic emotional responses, including blushing, pallor, sweating, dryness of the mouth, increased gastrointestinal motility, raised blood pressure and raised pulse rate.

5. *Sexual behaviour and reproduction.* Adenohypophysial gonadotrophin in part governs reproductive physiology. The limbic system mediates complex patterns of associated sexual behaviour such as identification of mate, home-building and care of offspring.

6. *Biological clocks.* There is a cyclical pattern, or *circadian rhythm*, in many tissues and functions. These are influenced by the hypothalamus, itself affected by diurnal rhythms. Based on twenty-four hours of light and darkness are cyclical patterns in body temperature, waking and sleeping, adrenocortical activity, renal secretion, plasma constituents, and eosinophil count. The most obvious example, the sleeping pattern, may be much disturbed by hypothalamic lesions.

APPLIED ANATOMY

The functional importance of the hypothalamus is disproportionate to its small size. Clinical features of its dysfunction are interesting and instructive and may follow trauma, inflammation, neoplastic compression or ischaemia. *Diabetes insipidus*, developing spontaneously or after head injury, involves impaired secretion of anti-diuretic hormone; the urine volume is very large, its specific gravity low; absence of glycosuria differentiates it from diabetes mellitus. Defective temperature regulation, resulting in *hyperthermia* or *hypothermia*, may follow head injury or local surgery. Traumatic anteroposterior displacement of the cerebral hemispheres distorts this region; following severe concussion there may be *somnolence* and '*cerebral irritation*' in which the patient curls up in bed, knees and arms flexed, verbally and physically resenting any interference. Similar '*sham rage*' can be evoked by experimental hypothalamic stimulation. *Fröhlich's syndrome* (dystrophia-adiposo-genitalis), which includes obesity, stunted growth and genital hypoplasia, may occur in children as a result of either a pituitary tumour or hypothalamic dysfunction. *Psychological response to altered endocrine balance* includes premenstrual tension, postpuerperal psychosis and menopausal emotional lability.

Chapter 9

Corpus striatum

Deep to the cortex in each cerebral hemisphere are masses of grey matter, collectively termed the *basal ganglia*. The largest is the *corpus striatum*, topographically divided into a *caudate nucleus* and a *lentiform nucleus*, the lentiform nucleus consisting of an outer *putamen* and inner *globus pallidus* (*Figs.* 9.1, 9.2). Between the putamen and the insular cortex is a thin grey sheet, the *claustrum*, of uncertain function. These masses form a motor complex which functionally includes the *substantia nigra* and the *subthalamic nucleus*. The amygdaloid nucleus has similar developmental origins but is functionally separate as part of the limbic system.

The major functional division of the corpus striatum is phylogenetic: the globus pallidus is relatively ancient and is termed the *paleostriatum*, or *pallidum*; the *neostriatum*, or *striatum* emerged in reptiles and comprises the caudate nucleus and the putamen, which are partially separated by the anterior limb of the internal capsule. The striatum is largely afferent, the pallidum efferent. These features may be summarized as follows:

$$\text{Corpus striatum} \begin{cases} \text{Paleostriatum (Pallidum)} &= \text{Globus pallidus} \\ \\ \text{Neostriatum (Striatum)} &= \begin{cases} \text{Putamen} \\ \text{Caudate nucleus} \end{cases} \end{cases} \Bigg\} \text{Lentiform nucleus}$$

TOPOGRAPHY

The *caudate nucleus* has an elongated curved tail (cauda) and is related throughout to the lateral ventricle. It has a large *head* bulging into the lateral wall of the anterior ventricular horn (*Fig.* 9.2). The anterior limb of the internal capsule partially separates the caudate head from the putamen of the lentiform nucleus, but numerous strands of grey matter connect them across the internal capsule; inferiorly the two structures are fused (*Fig.* 9.3). This fusion lies immediately above the anterior perforated substance which transmits the striate branches of the middle and anterior cerebral arteries. Near the interventricular foramen the head tapers rapidly into a narrow *body* in the lateral part of the ventricular floor, and a relatively slender *tail* curves down and then forwards in the roof of the inferior horn, with the amygdaloid nucleus at its tip. A bundle of fibres, the

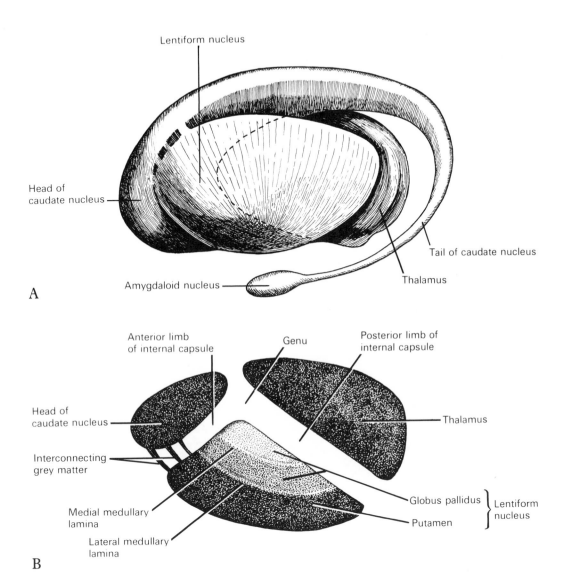

Fig. 9.1 The left corpus striatum and thalamus, (A) from the lateral aspect and (B) in horizontal section.

stria terminalis, leaves the amygdaloid nucleus and accompanies the medial edge of the caudate tail and body. In the floor of the central part of the ventricle, the stria terminalis and a *thalamostriate vein* lie between the caudate nucleus and the thalamus (*Figs.* 8.10, 14.6). The vein receives blood from the thalamus, corpus striatum and internal capsule.

The *lentiform nucleus* appears biconvex in some sections, cuneiform in others. Its lateral surface is gently convex and separated from the claustrum by the *external capsule*. Between the claustrum and insula is the *extreme capsule* (*Figs.* 9.2, 9.4). In transverse sections, the medial surface of the lentiform nucleus is angulated at the genu of the internal capsule, partly separated by the capsule's anterior limb from the caudate head and from the thalamus by its posterior limb. The inferior lentiform surface is deeply grooved by the anterior commissure (interconnecting the temporal lobes) and lies close to the anterior perforated substance. The nucleus is above structures in the roof of the inferior ventricular horn and the sublentiform part of the internal capsule (auditory

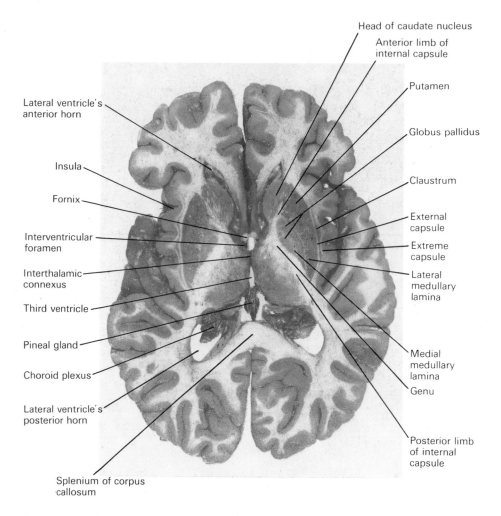

Fig. 9.2 Horizontal section of the cerebrum at the level of the interventricular foramina. (Mulligan's stain, 0.6 natural size.)

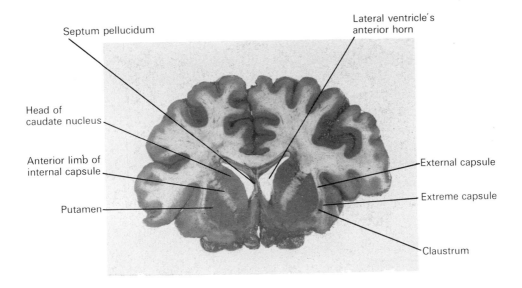

Fig. 9.3 Coronal section of the cerebrum through the anterior horns of the lateral ventricles. (Mulligan's stain, 0.6 natural size.)

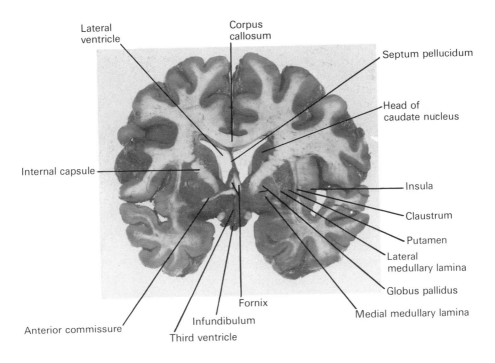

Fig. 9.4 Coronal section of the cerebrum at the level of the infundibulum. (Mulligan's stain, 0.6 natural size.)

radiation). The amygdaloid nucleus is situated below the lentiform nucleus at the inferior horn's tip.

In section the lentiform nucleus displays a dark external zone, the putamen, and a lighter internal part, the globus pallidus. The putamen is densely cellular and identical in structure to the caudate nucleus. The globus pallidus is traversed by many myelinated fasciculae giving it a pale colour. A thin lateral medullary lamina separates the putamen and the globus pallidus; a medial medullary lamina divides the globus pallidus into medial and lateral segments (*Figs.* 9.2, 9.4, 7.9).

STRIATAL CONNEXIONS

The *striatum* (caudate nucleus and putamen) is the receptive region of the corpus striatum; most of its output is to the globus pallidus (the pallidum). Some efferents also reach the substantia nigra.

Striatal afferent fibres

Afferents are received from the *cerebral cortex, thalamus* and *substantia nigra. Corticostriate* fibres are profuse and from most parts of the cerebral cortex, particularly the somatomotor region, and have a topographical arrangement. Thus the 'facial region' of the primary motor cortex projects to the ventral putamen, and the 'leg area' to its dorsal part. Corticofugal fibres enter the striatum via the internal and external capsules; they are not collaterals of the corticospinal and corticobulbar fibres but arise from a layer of small pyramidal cells in the external half of cortical lamina V. *Thalamostriate* fibres mostly start in the centromedian nucleus, and also in the smaller intralaminar nuclei and dorsal medial nucleus. *Nigrostriate* fibres, significant in relation to Parkinson's disease (characterized by tremor and muscular rigidity), utilize dopamine as a neurotransmitter and are inhibitory, possibly smoothing large peaks of striatal electrical discharge. *Brainstem* afferents from the raphé nuclei (in the periaqueductal grey matter) transport inhibitory serotonin to the striatum. (Nuclei of the raphé have been mentioned in relation to a descending pain control pathway).

Striatal efferent fibres

Most striatal efferents are *striatopallidal*, myelinated fibres passing to one of the segments of the globus pallidus. *Striatonigral* fibres mostly carry inhibitory GABA neurotransmitter to the substantia nigra, but some are excitatory and use substance P; these connexions are reciprocal to the nigrostriate fibres. Disease of the substantia nigra (*Fig.* 9.6) is usually explained primarily on the basis of its efferent, dopaminergic nigrostriate path, but the reciprocal relationship implies a more complex derangement.

PALLIDAL CONNEXIONS

As the main efferent striatal component, the globus pallidus receives most of the striatal output; it also has reciprocal connexions with the subthalamic nucleus.

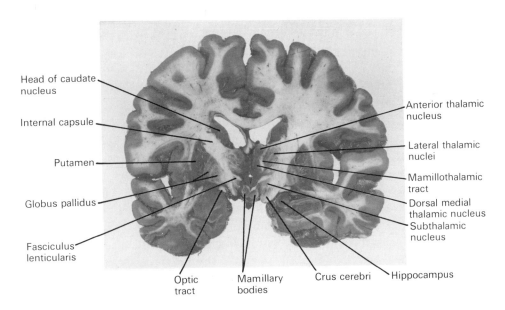

Fig. 9.5 Coronal section of the cerebrum at the level of the mamillary bodies. (Mulligan's stain, 0.6 natural size.)

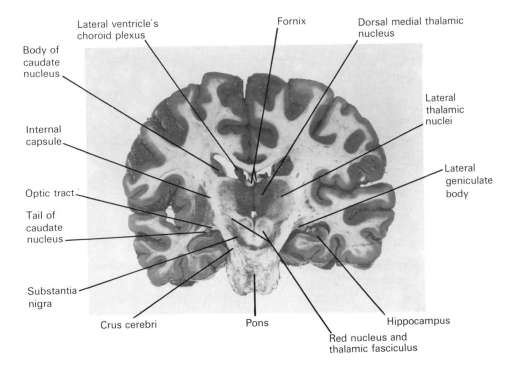

Fig. 9.6 Coronal section of the cerebrum through the thalami, crura cerebri and pons. (Mulligan's stain, 0.6 natural size.)

Pallidal efferents

Outflow from the globus pallidus is mainly to the thalamus. As previously noted, this is via two fasciculi; the *ansa lenticularis* looping round the posterior limb of the internal capsule and the *fasciculus lenticularis* traversing the internal capsule (*Figs.* 8.6, 9.5). These fasciculi enter the region between the red nucleus and the thalamus (prerubral field) to meet the dentato-rubro-thalamic tract and unite as the *thalamic fasciculus*. This leads to thalamic ventral lateral and ventral anterior nuclei, which project to the motor and premotor cortex. The corpus striatum influences descending pathways via this thalamocortical projection, also linked with cerebellar efferents.

The *subthalamic fasciculus* passes through the internal capsule to the subthalamic nucleus (*Figs.* 8.6, 8.9) and also conveys fibres from the nucleus to the globus pallidus. *Pallidonigral* efferents pass to the substantia nigra. A *pallidohabenular* connexion has been described which, through the habenular nucleus, may influence the limbic system. A small group of *pallidotegmental* fibres reach the lower midbrain, but there is no projection beyond this to the brainstem or the spinal cord.

FUNCTIONS OF THE BASAL GANGLIA

In sub-mammalian vertebrates, the diencephalon and corpus striatum are sensory and motor integrating and control centres, combined in the performance of stereotyped activity. In later evolution, the activities of the corpus striatum become subordinate to those of the cerebral cortex, but remain essential to muscle tone, quality of movement, posture and locomotion. The corpus striatum, substantia nigra and subthalamic nucleus are functionally interdependent. Disease in any part of this complex of extra-pyramidal nuclei upsets total function, and the symptoms reflect general derangement. Dysfunction of one component may result in over-activity in another part of the complex ('release phenomenon').

APPLIED ANATOMY

Diseases of the basal ganglia cause changes in muscle tone, postural disorders, and spontaneous involuntary movements. The latter take various forms: *tremors*; *athetosis* – uncontrolled writhing movements of the distal parts of limbs, particularly the hands and forearms; *chorea* – rapid, jerky, purposeless movements, often accompanied by grimacing and twitching of the facial muscles; *ballismus* – violent flailing limb movements at shoulder or hip.

Parkinson's disease is characterized by tremor, rigidity and slowness of movement. The hands tremble when the limb is at rest, unlike the 'intention tremor' of cerebellar disease which accompanies movement. Muscular rigidity, with slowness and general poverty of movement, results in a shuffling gait, stooped posture, slow speech and mask-like, emotionless face. The condition follows degeneration of dopamine-producing neurons in the substantia nigra and their nigrostriate axons, with a consequent absence of dopamine in the striatum (melanin, normally present in the substantia nigra, is a by-product of dopamine metabolism). Alleviation is by administration of L–dopa which, unlike dopamine, crosses the blood/brain barrier. Tremor and rigidity may be reduced by stereotactic surgery to place a small destructive lesion in the ventral lateral thalamic nucleus; this diminishes the cortical effects of abnormal discharges from the corpus striatum. Striatal implants of dopamine-containing neurons of foetal origin is effective experimentally in rats but is not applicable to human Parkinsonism; autograft implantation of dopamine cells from patients' adrenal glands is being evaluated in a Scandinavian centre.

Athetosis follows cerebral injury during birth, or congenital maldevelopment; it is accompanied by spasticity. Degeneration is usually found in the neostriatum and the adjacent cortex.

Sydenham's chorea, a disease of children, is associated with rheumatic fever; patients usually recover. Small haemorrhagic lesions in the corpus striatum have been described in fatal cases. *Huntington's chorea* is a hereditary disorder which usually appears in adult life and progresses to dementia. It is associated with degeneration of striatonigral GABA neurons, and intrastriatal cholinergic neurons. The loss of GABA-mediated control of the substantia nigra allows its dopaminergic neurons to inhibit striatal activity excessively.

Hemiballismus consists of violent, jerky, flinging movements of limbs contralateral to lesions in a subthalamic nucleus, usually the result of vascular occlusion. This disorder has been produced experimentally in monkeys by localized destruction in the subthalamic nucleus. It is much more difficult to mimic other disorders of the basal ganglia by experimental methods.

Chapter 10

Olfactory and limbic systems

In some vertebrates the olfactory sense is of primary importance, and the *rhinencephalon*, the olfactory part of the brain, is relatively large. In such *macrosmatic* animals it is related not only to searching for food, but also to mating, care and identification of offspring, danger, defence and offence. Man is *microsmatic*, with a much reduced olfaction: the rhinencephalon is relatively small and is overshadowed by the great development of the cerebral hemispheres. The olfactory cortex is small in area, wider emotional and behavioural reactions, originally associated with the rhinencephalon, being mediated by the limbic system.

OLFACTORY PATHWAYS

The olfactory epithelium occupies about one square inch in the nasal roof. It contains *bipolar neurons* whose peripheral processes have superficial ciliated receptors, sensitive to odiferous substances dissolved or suspended in the suprajacent mucus. Non-myelinated axons of these neurons form about twenty bundles of *olfactory nerves* which pierce the ethmoidal cribriform plates to terminate in each olfactory bulb, where they converge on *synaptic glomeruli*. There is further convergence to secondary sensory neurons, either *mitral cells* (shaped like a mitre) or smaller *tufted cells*, whose axons form the *olfactory tract*. Interneurons also occur in the bulb. The *anterior olfactory nucleus*, a small collection of cells at the junction of the bulb and the tract, has axons which cross to the opposite bulb in the anterior commissure. Posteriorly the olfactory tract divides into *medial and lateral olfactory striae* at the anterior perforated substance (*Fig.* 10.1); the lateral stria ends in the *primary olfactory cortex* of the uncus and part of the amygdaloid nucleus, communicating with the *olfactory association cortex* of the adjacent part of the parahippocampal gyrus. There are also connexions with the grey matter of the anterior perforated substance (perforated by striate arteries). The *diagonal stria* (of Broca) passes between the amygdaloid nucleus and the septal area, forming a caudal boundary to the anterior perforated substance. The medial olfactory stria projects to the *septal area*, located anterior to the lamina terminalis and inferior to the rostrum of the corpus callosum.

Reflex responses to olfaction, for example salivation and gastric secretion, are mediated by two autonomic pathways from the septal area to the brainstem: the *medial*

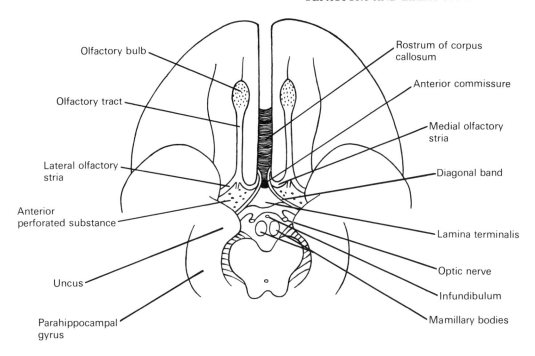

Fig. 10.1 Olfactory structures on the ventral surface of the brain. (The optic nerves have been retracted posteriorly.)

forebrain bundle traverses the lateral part of the hypothalamus; the *stria medullaris thalami* crosses the ventricular thalamic surface to the habenular nucleus (*Fig.* 8.10), where it relays to the interpeduncular nucleus of the midbrain. A further relay to the tegmentum forms the *dorsal longitudinal fasciculus* in the periaqueductal grey matter. Descending hypothalamic and limbic efferents also utilize these pathways.

APPLIED ANATOMY

Head injuries which involve anteroposterior movement of the brain may tear the olfactory nerves and cause permanent *anosmia*. The injured frequently complain also of loss of taste, since much of our interpretation of taste is related to olfactory stimuli. If a cribriform plate is fractured, cerebrospinal fluid may leak into the nose, and bacteria may enter, causing meningitis. *Uncinate fits* occur when epilepsy involves the temporal lobe: the 'aura' before an attack takes the form of olfactory hallucinations.

THE LIMBIC SYSTEM

The limbic system is so named because it occupies a bordering zone (limbus) between the diencephalon and telencephalon, and is functionally intermediate between the emotive and cognitive aspects of consciousness. Sensory input from the thalamus and

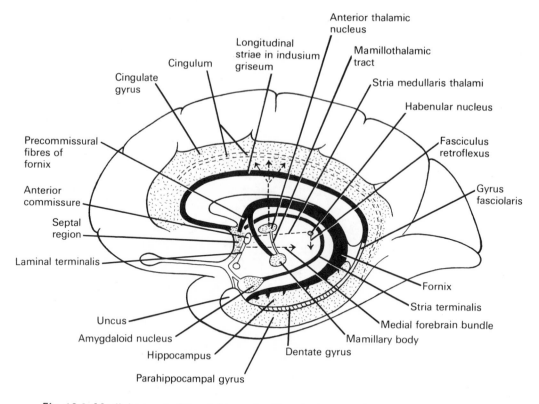

Fig. 10.2 Medial aspect of the right cerebral hemisphere to show structures included in the limbic system (stippled) and their tracts (black).

hypothalamus is processed here in regard to emotional and behavioural reactions which relate to the preservation of the individual and the species. Olfactory input is insignificant in man, but the limbic system appears important to memory.

The major limbic components (*Fig.* 10.2) are the *septal area, cingulate* and *parahippocampal gyri, hippocampal formation, amygdaloid nucleus, mamillary bodies* and *anterior thalamic nucleus.* Sparse grey matter on the upper surface of the corpus callosum, the *indusium griseum,* and in the septum pellucidum have developmental and phylogenetic significance (*Fig.* 1.7). Connecting limbic pathways include the *fornix, mamillothalamic tract, cingulum, stria terminalis* and *medial and lateral longitudinal striae.* Descending pathways are the *mamillotegmental tract, medial forebrain bundle* and *stria medullaris thalami.*

Many of these structures have a curvature determined by progressive development of the cerebral hemispheres, first posteriorly, then anteroinferiorly around the diencephalon. The hippocampus, a relatively ancient structure (archecortex), is located dorsally in reptiles and early mammals, curving over the anterior (olfactory) commissure from the septal area, a pattern also seen in the early stages of development of the human brain (*Fig.* 1.7). With the development of the cerebral hemispheres (neocortex) and corpus callosum, the hippocampus has been displaced downwards into the temporal lobe and rolled medially. The indusium griseum and longitudinal striae indicate the track of this displacement and provide a vestigial connexion in man between the hippocampus and the septal area.

Hippocampal formation

This comprises the *hippocampus, dentate gyrus* and *subiculum*. The subiculum is a transitional zone between the three-layered hippocampal archecortex and the six-layered neocortex of the parahippocampal gyrus.

The hippocampus (*Fig.* 10.3) is an area of cortex rolled into the floor of the inferior horn of the lateral ventricle, continuous medially with the subiculum and parahippocampal gyrus. The name 'hippocampus', meaning 'sea horse', is derived from its appearance in coronal section (*Fig.* 10.4). Its anterior extremity forms a paw-like *pes hippocampi*. On its ventricular surface is a layer of white matter, the *alveus*, whose fibres converge medially to a longitudinal ridge, the *fimbria of the fornix*. The choroid fissure and choroid plexus are above the fimbria. Posteriorly the hippocampus ends beneath the splenium of the corpus callosum.

The dentate gyrus, a serrated band of grey matter between the fimbria and subiculum, is overhung by the fimbria and is best viewed from the medial aspect. Anteriorly the

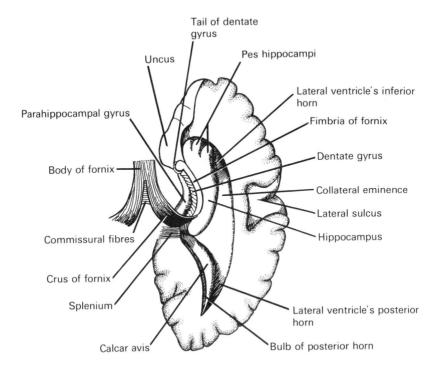

Fig. 10.3 A dissection of the inferior and posterior horns of the right lateral ventricle.

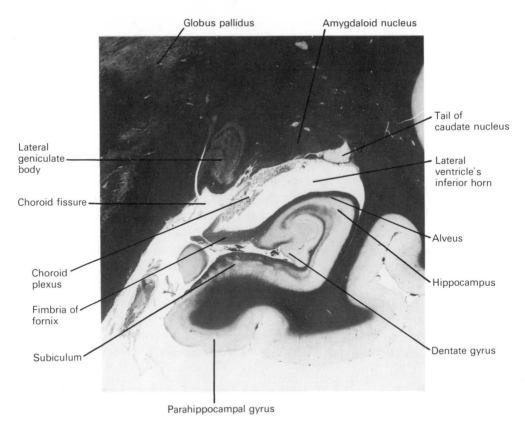

Fig. 10.4 Coronal section through the hippocampal formation. (Lithium haematoxylin and darrow red stain, × 3.5.)

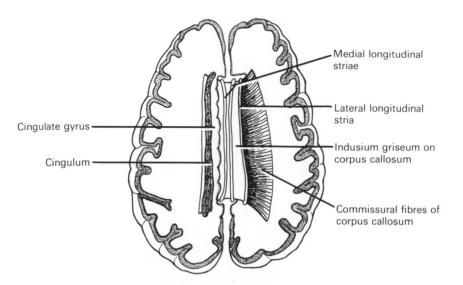

Fig. 10.5 Superior aspect of the corpus callosum. The cerebral hemispheres have been sectioned above the cingulate gyri, the left cingulate gyrus dissected to reveal the cingulum and the right cingulate gyrus removed and some callosal fibres shown.

dentate gyrus blends with the uncus; posteriorly it continues through the slender *gyrus fasciolaris* into the *indusium griseum*, the vestigial grey matter on the upper surface of the corpus callosum. The medial and lateral longitudinal striae, two narrow fasciculi embedded in the indusium griseum on each side, extend forwards to the septal area (*Fig.* 10.5).

The hippocampus has three neuronal layers termed the superficial molecular, middle pyramidal, and deep polymorphous layers. Axons of the pyramidal neurons pass through the alveus into the fornix. The dentate gyrus is also trilaminar, but its middle layer is of granular cells.

Connexions of the hippocampal formation (*Figs.* 10.2, 10.6)

The fornix receives fibres from the hippocampus and subiculum. Posteriorly the fimbriae form *crura* curving over the thalamus and united above in the *body* of the fornix. A transverse *hippocampal commissure* between the crura interconnects the two hippocampi. The body of the fornix is closely related to the corpus callosum above and separated below from the thalami by the choroid fissures. Anteriorly, the body of the fornix divides into two *columns* which arch down towards the anterior commissure, and form the anterior boundary of the interventricular foramen on each side. The columns of the fornix traverse the hypothalamus and end in the *mamillary bodies*. Each mamillo-

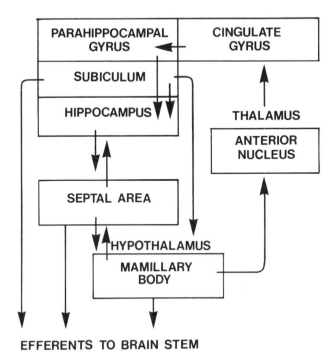

Fig. 10.6 Schematic diagram of some major components in the limbic system. The amygdaloid nucleus is excluded.

thalamic tract has reciprocal connexions with its *anterior thalamic nucleus*, which projects to the ipsilateral cingulate gyrus. Within the gyrus, a bundle of myelinated fibres, the *cingulum*, curves posteroinferiorly into the *parahippocampal gyrus*, providing an input to the hippocampus through the subiculum. This path is sometimes dubbed the 'Papez circuit', after the neuroanatomist who described it in 1937 as having possible significance in emotional disorders. The human hippocampus is no longer part of the olfactory system.

The fornix projects to the *septal area* through a *precommissural fasciculus*. Another connexion from the fornix to the septal area is via fibres in the *longitudinal striae* above the corpus callosum. The hippocampus also receives a feedback from the septal area via the fornix and longitudinal striae.

Amygdaloid nucleus

This almond-shaped mass is anterosuperior to the tip of the lateral ventricle's inferior horn. It has already been noted that part of it has an olfactory input. Its larger, ventrolateral part is included in the limbic system and has complex cortical, thalamic and hypothalamic afferents. Its main efferent tract is the *stria terminalis*, which runs posteriorly in the roof of the inferior horn, medial to the tail of the caudate nucleus, and curves into the floor of the body of the lateral ventricle, where it lies between the caudate nucleus and the thalamus. It projects to the septal area, anterior hypothalamus and habenular nucleus.

Limbic projections to the brainstem

There are three paths by which the limbic system influences autonomic centres in the brainstem: (1) the medial forebrain bundle, from the septal area and hypothalamus; (2) the stria medullaris thalami, to the habenular nucleus and via the fasciculus retroflexus to the interpeduncular nucleus, thence to the dorsal longitudinal fasciculus; (3) the mamillotegmental tract. These have already been mentioned.

Functions of the limbic system

Ablation or stimulation of parts of the limbic system produces various behavioural and emotional changes, in general related to *preservation of the individual or the species*. Individual responses to a challenging situation may involve offensive or defensive reactions, anger, fear and acceleration of heart and of respiration. Species preservation includes sexual responses, mating and the care of offspring. There are so-called '*pleasure centres*' in the limbic system. Thus, if a human septal area is stimulated by an electrode under local anaesthesia, the patient feels happy, is less inhibited and more talkative.

The limbic system participates in a *memory retention mechanism*. Lesions of the temporal lobe involving the hippocampus depress memorization of recent events, although long-established memories are unaffected. Details of this mechanism are uncertain. As noted previously, the anterior and dorsal medial thalamic nuclei also play a role in memorization.

APPLIED ANATOMY

Bilateral removal of anterior parts of the temporal lobes, either experimentally or in the treatment of severe epilepsy originating here, results in the *Klüver-Bucy syndrome*, characterized by increased appetite, loss of recent memories, docility and hyper-sexuality, the latter not necessarily heterosexual.

Experimental stimulation of the *amygdaloid nuclei* produces excitability, fear and rage; stereotactic surgical lesions have been used clinically to reduce pathological aggression in certain cases.

Following *Wernicke's encephalopathy*, a vitamin deficiency associated with alcoholism, there is a permanent memory loss, sometimes attributed to the haemorrhage and atrophy found in the mamillary bodies.

Temporal lobe epilepsy has been mentioned in connexion with olfactory hallucinations. Other symptoms such as altered awareness of surroundings, bizarre behaviour, temporary amnesia and unusual visceral sensations may be due to limbic dysfunction.

Chapter 11

Visual system

The optic nerve and retina develop from an outgrowth of the forebrain vesicle. Near the skin this outgrowth invaginates as a bilaminar optic cup, the outer layer becoming the black pigmented retinal epithelium, the inner forming the neural retinal layers. These two basic laminae are closely apposed, but may separate in the clinical condition, 'detached retina'.

THE RETINA

From within outwards (i.e. from vitreous to choroid) the retina consists of *nerve fibres*, *ganglion cells*, *bipolar cells*, *photoreceptors* and *pigment epithelium*, with supportive neuroglial cells (*Fig*. 11.1). The nerve fibres converge to the *optic disc*, slightly medial to the posterior ocular pole, pierce the sclera, become myelinated and form the optic nerve. The optic disc is insensitive to light and hence is known as the 'blind spot'. The central retinal artery and vein also traverse the disc. Immediately lateral to the disc and in line with the visual axis is the oval, slightly yellow *macula lutea*, which has a central depression, the *fovea centralis*, where visual acuity is maximal; there are no nerve fibres or blood vessels in front of it. In purposeful vision the eyes are directed so that the retinal image is on the macula lutea.

The *pigment epithelium* contains melanin which absorbs light and prevents back-scatter. Its external aspect is firmly attached to the choroid; its internal surface is infolded between individual photoreceptors. The *photoreceptors*, rods and cones, have an external light-sensitive segment containing photopigments, a cell body and a synaptic base. They transduce light into electrical energy. *Rods* are more numerous than cones, contain the pigment rhodopsin (visual purple), and are most sensitive in conditions of low illumination, for example at night. The fovea is 'night-blind' because it contains no rods. *Cones* are more discriminative of detail and sensitive to colour; each contains one of three pigments sensitive to blue, green or red light. Perception of colour requires a neural interaction between the cones to correlate the trichromatic input. Cones predominate in the macula lutea and diminish rapidly away from it; only cones are present in the central fovea.

In the retina (*Fig*. 11.1) there is direct neuronal transmission from the photoreceptors via bipolar cells and ganglion cells, and also a lateral interacting system of interneurons

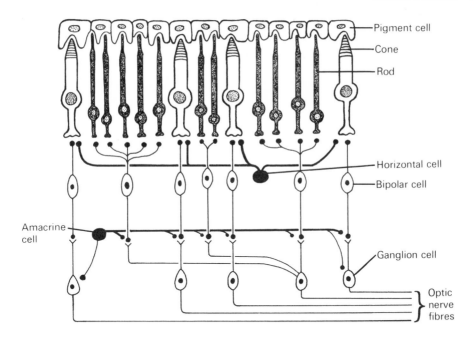

Fig. 11.1 Neuronal pathways in the retina.

(horizontal cells and amacrine cells), whereby visual information is modulated and integrated. Transmission is either convergent (rods) or relatively non-convergent and more discriminative (cones). Large numbers of rods synapse with one bipolar cell, many of which converge to one ganglion cell. This summation contributes to sensitivity of the rod system in poor lighting, but limits discrimination. There is little such convergence among cones, and foveal cones have a 1 : 1 : 1 ratio with their bipolar and ganglion cells, thus ensuring high resolution. Axons from the ganglion cells form the optic nerve. Retinal nerve fibres are non-myelinated, an optical advantage since myelin is highly refractile.

VISUAL PATHWAY

The two *optic nerves* extend from the eyes to the optic chiasma, each containing about one million axons, myelinated by oligodendrocytes, and surrounded by pia mater, arachnoid mater and dura mater. Pia mater invests the nerve and is separated from the arachnoid mater by a subarachnoid space. The central retinal vessels traverse this space, and if the cerebrospinal fluid pressure is abnormally raised, the vein is compressed, with resultant oedema of the optic disc (papilloedema). The dural sleeve fuses with the ocular sclera. At the optic chiasma, fibres derived from the nasal half of each retina cross. Some crossed fibres loop forward slightly into the contralateral optic nerve before entering the optic tract; some loop backwards into the ipsilateral tract before crossing (*Fig.* 11.5). Each *optic tract* extends from the chiasma to the lateral geniculate body, where most of

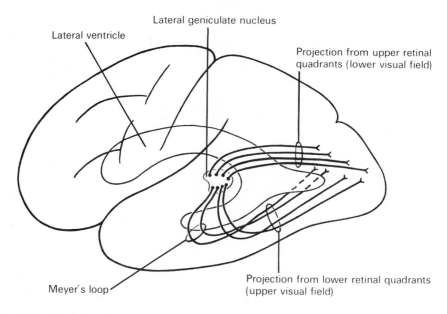

Fig. 11.2 The left optic radiation viewed from the lateral aspect.

its fibres end. A few fibres leave each optic tract to descend in a *superior brachium* to the ipsilateral superior colliculus and both pretectal nuclei. These mesencephalic connexions respectively subserve reflex neck movements (such as turning the head towards a flash of light) and the pupillary light reflex. The *optic radiation* (geniculo-calcarine tract) is in the retrolentiform part of the internal capsule. Fibres passing to the primary visual cortex above the calcarine sulcus fan out round the lateral ventricle's posterior horn; fibres passing to the visual cortex below the sulcus loop down into the temporal lobe, lateral to the ventricle's inferior horn (Meyer's loop) (*Fig.* 11.2). The optic radiation also includes fibres descending <u>*from*</u> the occipital cortex to the superior colliculus via the superior brachium.

The *primary visual cortex* (area 17 of Brodmann) is also known as the striate cortex, because section reveals a horizontal *visual stria* (of Gennari) in its grey matter (*Fig.* 12.5). The *visual association cortex* (Brodmann areas 18, 19) occupies the remaining areas of the occipital lobe and is concerned with complex aspects of visual perception; it receives fibres from the thalamic pulvinar and is the source of corticocollicular fibres mediating the pupillary accommodation reflex, visual grasp reflex and automatic scanning.

IMAGE PROJECTION AND PROCESSING

Light from the left half of the visual field impinges on the right halves of the two retinae, which project to the right visual cortex. The cornea and lens produce a retinal image which is inverted and reversed (left to right), and this pattern is transferred to the visual cortex. As illustrated in *Fig.* 11.3, a sequential cortical projection requires decussation of the optic nerves. In the panoramic vision of sub-mammalian vertebrates there is total decussation. In human binocular vision half the fibres decussate: the resultant fusion of images viewed from a slightly different angle by each eye produces stereoscopic perception of depth and distance. Commissural fibres in the corpus callosum are said to interconnect the occipital lobes to correlate the right and left visual fields.

There is very accurate point-to-point projection from the retina, in the visual pathway, to the visual cortex. *Fig.* 11.4 shows that the lower retinal quadrants are connected laterally in the ipsilateral geniculate body and project to the visual cortex *below* the calcarine sulcus. The upper retinal quadrants project to the medial part of their lateral geniculate bodies and to the visual cortex *above* the sulcus. There is a

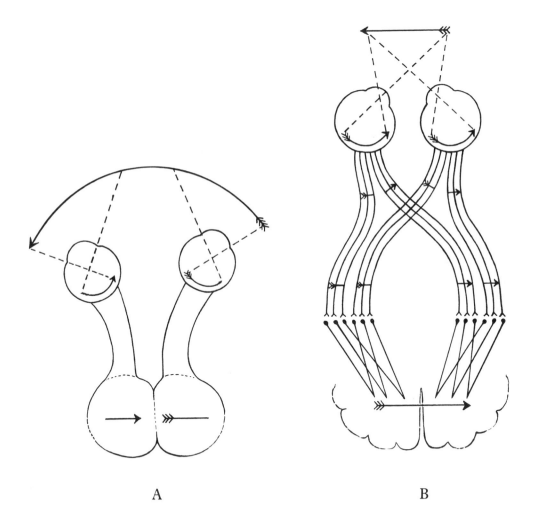

A   B

Fig. 11.3 Image projection in visual pathways. In the hypothetical condition (A), with no decussation of optic nerves, central projection of the image would be illogical. In man (B) half the optic nerve fibres decussate; image projection is sequentially reconstructed in pathways to visual cortex. (After Sarnat H. B. and Netsky M. G. (1974) *Evolution of the Nervous System.* Oxford, Oxford University Press.)

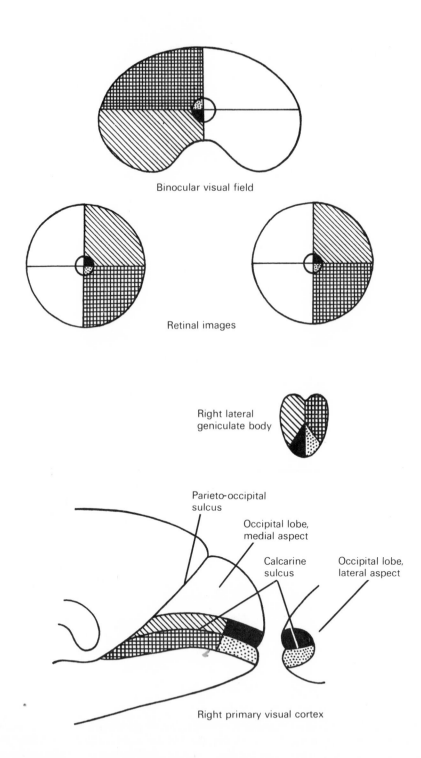

Fig. 11.4 Representation of the visual fields in the retinae, right lateral geniculate body and visual cortex.

disproportionately large macular representation in the geniculate bodies and in the posterior third of the primary visual cortices. This accords with the macula's functional importance; the number of fibres from the macular ganglion cells is large because of the discrete, non-convergent projection from its photoreceptors.

Each *lateral geniculate body* has six layers of neurons, numbered 1–6 from the ventral to the dorsal surface. Crossed optic fibres terminate in layers 1, 4 and 6, uncrossed optic fibres in layers 2, 3 and 5. It is not simply a relay station: in each lamina are interneurons which further integrate visual impulses, but there is little exchange between laminae.

The lateral geniculate axons terminate primarily in the visual stria (of Gennari), which is in layer IV (*see* Chapter 12) of the *visual cortex*. From each of the six laminae of a lateral geniculate body the input is either from the right or the left eye. Cortical layers above and below layer IV effect binocular integration. Hubel and Wiesel (1974) showed that visual cortical neurons are organized into narrow columns extending from the cortical surface to the central white matter. Whereas geniculate cells respond to spots of light shone on the retina, these cortical neurons react to lines and edges; each column reacts to only one orientation of an image, that is vertical or at a particular angle to it. They are hence dubbed *orientation columns*. Also, since they receive an input from only one eye, they are grouped into larger *ocular dominance columns*. The visual cortex contains alternating right and left ocular dominance columns, each of which represents a complete series of orientation columns covering a 180° pattern of linear excitation in the visual field. This regular arrangement of the cortical ocular dominance columns is only partially developed at birth; full development depends on subsequent binocular excitation. Deprivation of input from one eye in the neonatal period results in irreversible cortical change, an imbalance in the size of left-right columns and permanent loss of normal binocular vision. This is an example of *neuronal plasticity*, in which cells of the stimulated column expand connexions into the adjacent quiescent area (Hubel, Wiesel and LeVay, 1977). It has obvious practical implications in the management of the newborn.

APPLIED ANATOMY

Visual defects may be mapped in detail by using an instrument called a perimeter. Gross defects can be detected by the confrontation method. The subject faces the examiner, eye to eye, and the latter moves an object, mid-way between himself and the subject, from the periphery towards the visual field and from differing directions. In each test the subject states when the object enters his visual field, and the examiner compares this rough estimate of the field with his own perceptions.

Lesions of the visual pathway are illustrated in *Fig.* 11.5. Defects are usually described in terms of the loss of visual fields. Loss of half a visual field of one or both eyes is *hemianopia*. Damage of one optic nerve (1) results in monocular blindness. A pituitary tumour may compress decussating fibres in the optic chiasma (2), causing bitemporal hemianopia. Pressure at the lateral edge of the optic chiasma (3) results in ipsilateral nasal hemianopia; if this is due to aneurysm of the internal carotid artery in the cavernous sinus, there will be a variable concomitant paralysis of eye muscles (ophthalmoplegia) due to compression of cranial nerves III, IV and VI. A lesion of the right optic

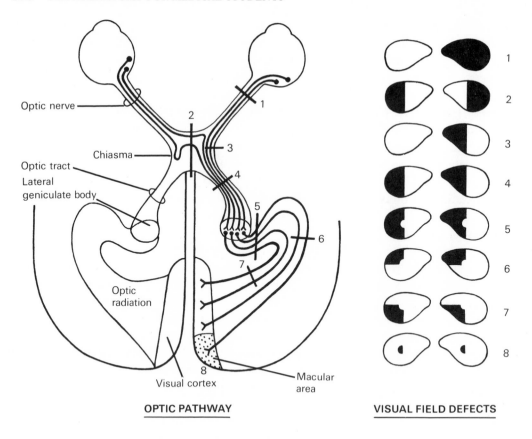

Optic nerve

Chiasma

Optic tract

Lateral
geniculate body

Optic
radiation

Optic
radiation

Visual cortex

Macular
area

OPTIC PATHWAY

VISUAL FIELD DEFECTS

Fig. 11.5 Visual field defects in lesions of the visual pathway (*see* text).

tract (4) produces a left homonymous hemianopia, that is loss of the same half of the visual field of both eyes. A complete lesion of the optic radiation (5) has a similar effect but, because the radiation fans out, partial or *quadrantic* defects are more common (6, 7). In field defects due to damage by posterior cerebral artery thrombosis there is often 'macular sparing' since a branch of the middle cerebral artery also reaches the macular area of the primary visual cortex (5, 6, 7). Damage of the cerebral occipital pole, often due to trauma, may destroy the macular area, producing a *central scotoma* (8).

Chapter 12

Cerebral cortex

CYTOLOGY AND CYTOARCHITECTURE

The external cerebral surface is a grey mantle (pallium) of approximately 14 000 million neurons and accompanying neuroglia. Its total area, more than two square feet, is folded into gyri and sulci. The cortical depth, greater over the gyri, less in the sulci, varies from 4 mm in the precentral gyrus to 1.5 mm in the primary visual area. It reaches maximum size in about eight years, increasing thereafter only in synaptic complexity.

Primitively the cortex served olfaction, with only three cell layers; such rhinencephalic derivatives – *archecortex* (hippocampus, dentate gyrus) and *paleocortex* (olfactory) – are trilaminar (*see* p. 172). The *neocortex*, comprising 90% of the total human cortex, is six-layered. The cingulate gyrus, intermediate histologically and functionally and part of the limbic system, is *mesocortex*.

Cortical neurons

Golgi Type I neurons, with long axons, are either *pyramidal* or *fusiform*. Golgi Type II neurons, with short axons, are either *stellate* (granular), *horizontal* neurons (of Cajal) or *Martinotti* neurons (with ascending axons) (*Fig.* 12.1).

The *pyramidal neurons* have cell bodies which vary in height from 10 μm to 120 μm; the latter, the *giant pyramidal cells* (of Betz), occur in the motor cortex. Pyramidal cell apices, directed towards the surface, have *apical dendrites*, the *basal dendrites* are spread laterally, and all have *dendritic spines*; their axons emerge basally and mostly enter the white matter as *projection fibres* (to the spinal cord, brainstem, basal ganglia and diencephalon), as *commissural fibres* (interhemispheric) and as *association fibres* (intra-hemispheric). Some small, superficially placed, pyramidal cells have short axons passing only to deeper laminae. Their axons commonly have intracortical collateral branches. The small pyramidal cells are found mostly in lamina III, the large ones in lamina V.

Fusiform neurons are like pyramidal cells, with long apical dendrites directed to the surface, short basal dendrites, and projection, commissural and association axons; however, the somata which are in lamina VI are spindle shaped, with their long axes vertical to the surface.

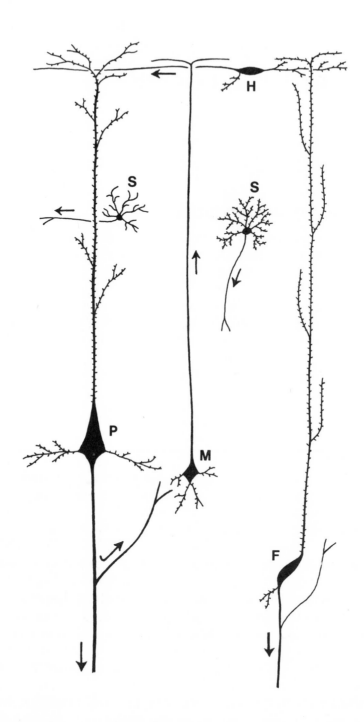

Fig. 12.1 Cortical neurons. **H**, horizontal neuron (of Cajal); **S**, stellate neuron; **P**, pyramidal neuron; **M**, Martinotti neuron; **F**, fusiform neuron.

Stellate neurons (granule cells) are concentrated in laminae II and IV, but are present throughout the cortex, except in the molecular lamina I. They have small, 8–10 μm star-shaped somata, with short axons and many dendrites.

Neurons of Martinotti, polygonal cells with short dendrites, have axons directed <u>towards</u> and often into lamina I, giving off collaterals en route. They occur in all laminae, except I.

Horizontal neurons (of Cajal) have small, fusiform somata, a dendrite at each pole and a longer axon, all parallel to the surface and restricted to lamina I. Obvious in the newborn, they are sparse in adults.

Laminar structure of the neocortex (*Figs.* 12.2, 12.3)

Regional cortical variations will be described later; the general pattern and functional attributes of the six-layered neocortex are:

I. *Molecular lamina.* The most superficial lamina, this is a synaptic field with few cells and many fine nerve fibres, including dendrites of pyramidal and fusiform neurons and axons of Martinotti neurons.

II. *External granular lamina.* Involved with *intracortical circuits* are large numbers of stellate and small pyramidal neurons with dendrites entering lamina I and axons directed to deeper laminae.

III. *External pyramidal lamina.* Concerned with *association and commissural* efferents, this contains medium-sized pyramidal cells superficially and larger ones more deeply, mingled with stellate and Martinotti neurons.

IV. *Internal granular lamina.* Receptive of *specific thalamic afferents* (e.g. from the geniculate or ventral posterior nuclei), this is a concentration of stellate neurons. In contrast to non-specific thalamic (e.g. reticular) and association afferents, which diffuse through all layers, the specific afferents have a bushy pattern of terminal fibres (*Fig.* 12.2): together with the fibres of stellate neurons these aggregate horizontally in this lamina as the outer band of Baillarger, a marked feature of the primary visual area, hence the name 'striate cortex' (*Fig.* 12.5).

V. *Inner pyramidal lamina.* This is a *source of major efferents* and is characterized by the presence of medium and large pyramidal neurons, including Betz cells. The latter contribute 3% of the corticospinal and corticobulbar fibres. Axon collaterals form the *inner band of Baillarger* in the deep part of this lamina (*Fig.* 12.4). Stellate and Martinotti neurons also occur.

VI. *Multiform lamina.* This is also an efferent lamina with neurons of various forms, many fusiform. Martinotti neurons are often numerous. This lamina mingles with the white matter, being pervaded by fibre bundles entering or leaving the cortex (*Fig.* 12.3A).

In identifying these laminae, first note the outer and inner bands of Baillarger in the middle of lamina IV and the deep part of lamina V respectively; secondly observe that laminae I and II are relatively narrow, lamina III very wide. Vertical intracortical fibres include dendrites and axons of pyramidal neurons and the axons of Martinotti neurons.

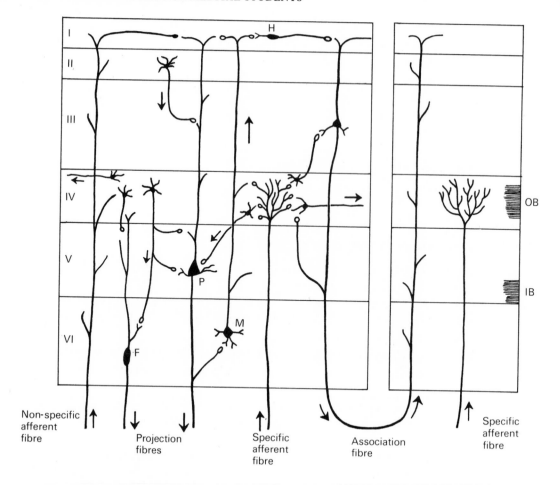

Fig. 12.2 A simplified diagram of intracortical circuits. **OB, IB**, outer and inner bands of Baillarger; **H, P, M, F** as in *Fig.* 12.1; laminae of the cortex are numbered I–VI.

Cortical classification

Homotypical cortex, in which all six layers are evident, occurs in 'association areas' (*see* functional localization). There are regional variations. The visual association cortex has pyramidal-type 'solitary cells' (of Meynert), the origin of corticocollicular fibres. The primary sensory and motor cortices are *heterotypical*: a six-layered pattern is obscured by the blending of laminae II–V, with a predominance of either stellate (sensory) or pyramidal (motor) neurons. The primary visual and auditory areas and the anterior part of the postcentral gyrus (Brodmann area 3) have a *granular cortex* with many stellate but few pyramidal neurons in laminae II–V. The precentral (motor) area has an *agranular cortex*: pyramidal neurons spread through layers II–V. *Allocortex*, of three layers, includes arche- and paleocortex; it is described in Chapter 10.

Brodmann (1909) classified the cortical areas in a cytoarchitectural map, based on a study of sub-human primate brains; fifty-seven areas were numbered. Though still

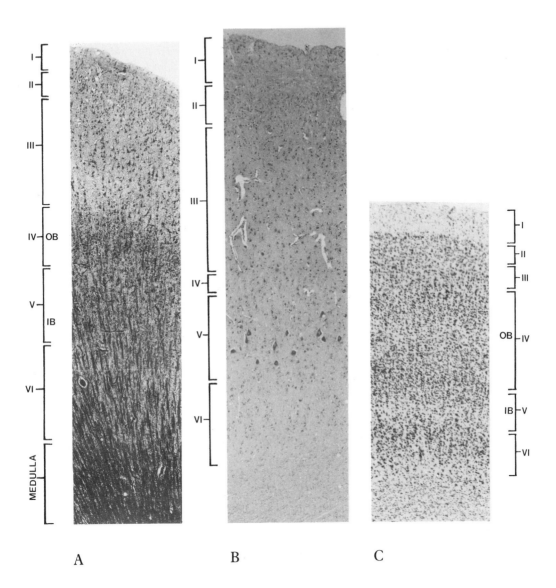

Fig. 12.3 Sections showing cortical structure, homotypical and heterotypical. Some dissimilarities are due to different staining methods. In the frontal cortex (A) myelinated fibres and cells are stained (Lithium haematoxylin and darrow red). In the motor cortex (B) and sensory cortex (C) only the cells are stained (by cresyl violet and toluidine blue respectively). Identify the inner (**IB**) and outer (**OB**) bands of Baillarger. Laminae of the cortex are numbered I–VI. (× *c.* 32, photographs by J. A. Findlay.)

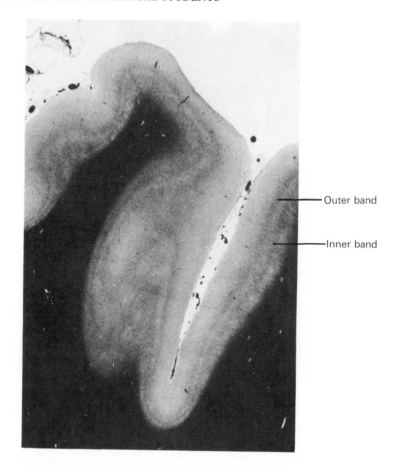

Outer band

Inner band

Fig. 12.4 Section showing bands of Baillarger in the frontal (homotypical) cortex. (Lithium haematoxylin and darrow red stain, × 6.)

widely used, such a division, with functional attributes, is over-precise. Even a basic division into 'motor' and 'sensory' areas is too rigid; for example some corticospinal fibres originate from the parietal 'sensory' cortex.

Functional columnar organization

In the receptive areas of the cortex, neuronal circuits are arranged in vertical columns. The neurons in each column have a common receptive field, respond to the same stimuli and discharge similarly. This is evident in the orientation columns and ocular dominance columns of the visual cortex (Chapter 11). Each column has its own afferent, efferent and internuncial fibres. The human cortex excels in its multitudinous stellate neurons, which form complex vertical interlaminar circuits and also link adjacent columns.

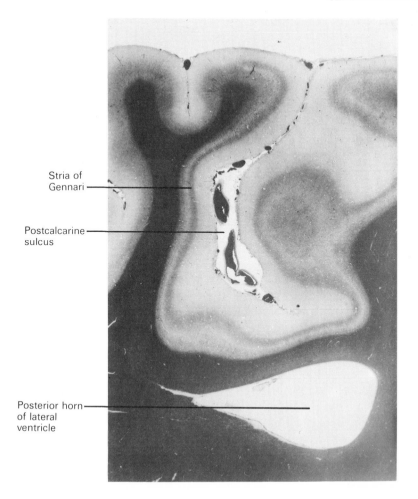

Fig. 12.5 A section of primary visual cortex. Note the stria of Gennari in both walls of the postcalcarine sulcus. The lateral ventricle's posterior horn has also been sectioned. (Lithium haematoxylin and darrow red stain, × 5.)

CEREBRAL WHITE MATTER

This is a compact mass of vast numbers of association, commissural and projection fibres and associated neuroglia.

Association fibres (*Fig.* 12.6).

Fibres interconnecting the cortical fibres in one hemisphere vary in length. *Short association fibres* link adjacent gyri. *Long association fibres* reciprocally connect different lobes. The *cingulum*, in the cingulate gyrus, is a limbic association bundle between the septal area and the parahippocampal gyrus. The *uncinate fasciculus*, originating in the motor

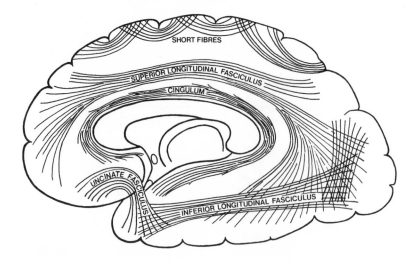

Fig. 12.6 The principal association fibres in the cerebrum.

speech area and the frontal lobe's orbital surface, hooks round the lateral fissure to reach the cortex at the temporal pole. The extensive *superior longitudinal fasciculus*, connecting the frontal and occipital poles, curves into the temporal lobe, receiving and giving off fibres en route. The *fronto-occipital fasciculus* pursues a similar course but is more deeply placed, separated from the superior longitudinal fasciculus by the corona radiata. The *inferior longitudinal fasciculus* connects the visual association area with the temporal lobe.

Commissural fibres

These join corresponding sites in the two hemispheres. Neocortical commissures are in the *corpus callosum* and the much smaller *anterior commissure*. Others are *habenular* (between the habenular nuclei), *hippocampal* (between the crura of the fornix) and *posterior commissural* (between the superior colliculi and the pretectal regions).

The *corpus callosum* is a massive, arched, interhemispheric bridge flooring the midline longitudinal fissure and roofing both lateral ventricles. It has a thin superficial grey mantle, the *indusium griseum*, embedded in which are white fibres of the bilateral *medial and lateral longitudinal striae*. The anterior cerebral vessels run in its pia mater. It is overhung by the median *falx cerebri* and overlapped laterally by the cingulate gyri. It is described as having a rostrum, genu, trunk and splenium (*Figs*. 8.1, 12.7). The curved anterior *genu* extends as a thin *rostrum* to the lamina terminalis. The *trunk*, the main body, ends posteriorly as a thickened *splenium* which overhangs the thalamic pulvinars, the pineal gland and the midbrain tectum. The *septum pellucidum* is a thin median sheet of white and grey matter, covered by ependyma and continuous with deep aspects of the rostrum, genu and anterior part of the trunk of the corpus callosum; posteriorly the trunk fuses with the body of the fornix. A *transverse fissure*, containing the tela choroidea of the third ventricle, posterior choroidal arteries and great cerebral vein, is inferior to

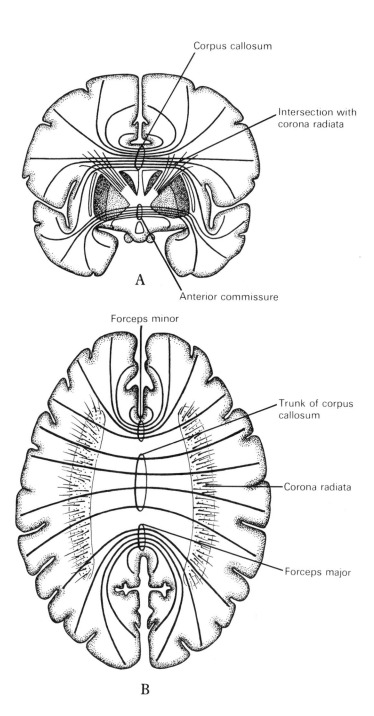

Corpus callosum

Intersection with
corona radiata

A

Anterior commissure

Forceps minor

Trunk of corpus
callosum

Corona radiata

Forceps major

B

Fig. 12.7 Interhemispheric (commissural) cortical connexions. (A) Coronal section
through the anterior commissure and corpus callosum. (B) Transverse section through
the corpus callosum.

the splenium. Callosal fibres traverse the medullary centres of the hemispheres to reach the cortex. Rostral fibres interconnect the orbital surfaces of the frontal lobes. Fibres in the genu radiate forwards as the *forceps minor* to the medial and lateral surfaces of the frontal lobes. Fibres in the callosal trunk pass laterally to extensive areas of the cortex, intersecting the corona radiata en route. Fibres to the temporal and inferior parts of the occipital lobes form a thin lamina, the *tapetum*, applied to the ependyma of the roof and lateral walls of each posterior horn, and to the lateral walls of each inferior horn of the lateral ventricles. A *forceps major* curves posteriorly from the splenium into both occipital lobes above the calcarine sulci, forming a *bulb of the posterior horn* in each lateral ventricle, bulging into its medial wall (*Fig.* 10.3).

The *anterior commissure* crosses as an oval bundle in the upper lamina terminalis, immediately in front of the anterior columns of the fornix. Its anterior fibres enter the anterior perforated substance and olfactory tract; posterior fibres form a fasciculus which deeply grooves the inferior aspects of the lentiform nuclei en route to anterior regions of the temporal lobes, including the parahippocampal gyri.

Commissural fibres are essential for the interhemispheric transfer of information for bilateral responses and in learning processes. The primary visual cortex and the 'hand area' of the primary somatosensory cortex have no known direct commissural fibres, but are abundantly correlated via the association areas. Severance of the corpus callosum in young monkeys causes a 'split brain' effect: trained to perform a task with one fore-paw, they are unable to replicate the act with the other paw. Section of the optic chiasma and splenium prevents the interchange of visual information between hemispheres.

Projection fibres

Corticofugal fibres project to the spinal cord, brainstem and diencephalon as cortico-spinal, corticobulbar, extrapyramidal (corticostriate, corticorubral, cortico-olivary, corticoreticular, corticonigral), corticopontine, corticothalamic and hypothalamic connexions. *Corticopetal* fibres relay from the thalamus to the cortex, except for an olfactory input. Almost all efferent fibres traverse the internal capsule; some cortico-striate fibres enter the external capsule; thalamocortical fibres ascend *into* the internal capsule. Between the internal capsule and the cortex fibres diverge as the *corona radiata*.

FUNCTIONAL LOCALIZATION

As already noted, the cerebral cortex is not divided into exclusively somatomotor and somatosensory regions. The pre- and postcentral areas are *both* sensorimotor, the former predominantly motor, the latter mostly sensory. There are supplementary somatomotor and somatosensory areas. The *relative* significance of these functional attributes can be expressed in an abbreviated form as follows: Precentral somato-motor = Ms I, supplementary somatomotor = Ms II, primary somatosensory = Sm I, supplementary somatosensory = Sm II. There are also visual and auditory primary sensory areas. Almost all the cortex supplies corticopontine fibres (from pyramidal neurons in the outer part of lamina V), which relay to the cerebellum.

'Primary' motor and sensory areas comprise only 14% of the human cortex, although much more in lower vertebrates (89% in the rat). The cortex can be regarded as consisting of two main types, 'primary' motor and sensory areas (mostly heterotypical in structure) and association areas (homotypical); but this is merely a convenient simplification of its complexities. The association areas have increased relatively throughout evolution to reach their summit in the human brain. Much of our understanding of such areas derives from clinical investigation of localized cortical injury. The diverse functions of the association areas include the interpretation of sensory input in relation to experience, the correlation of differing modalities (e.g. visual and auditory), complex behavioural responses and all 'thought'.

Parietal lobe

The *primary somatosensory area*, Sm I, occupies the *postcentral gyrus*, extending to the medial surface of the *posterior part of the paracentral lobule* (*Fig*. 12.8); it receives input from the ventral posterior thalamic nucleus. Histologically there are three narrow strips of cortex (Brodmann areas 3, 1, 2); area 3, in the posterior wall of the central sulcus, has a granular heterotypical structure and responds to tactile stimuli; areas 1 and 2 have a six-layered homotypical structure, and react to deep stimuli and joint movement. Nociceptive (pain or thermal) sensation reaches consciousness at thalamic level, but its qualitative and spatial evaluation is cortical. Gustatory impulses are received in the junctional region of the postcentral gyrus and insula. The area of cortex concerned with bodily regions is related to their functional skill and density of innervation rather than to size; the areas representing the mouth, face, eye and hand are disproportionally large (*Fig*. 12.9). The body image is inverted: the pharynx, tongue and jaws are most ventral, followed by the face, hand, arm and trunk; the lower limb, anal and genital regions are medial in the paracentral lobule. Most impulses are contralateral, although some from the oral region are ipsilateral and those from the pharynx, larynx and perineum project bilaterally. Localization is very discrete, for example individual vibrissae of the rodent muzzle are represented in vertically ordered 'barrel units'.

The *second somatosensory area*, Sm II, is in the superior lip of the lateral fissure, with the face anterior and the lower limb posterior. It has reciprocal connexions with Sm I and the thalamus, some being bilateral. Its functional significance is uncertain.

Somatosensory association area

The *superior parietal lobule* (Brodmann areas 5, 7) has reciprocal connexions with Sm I and with the dorsal tier of lateral thalamic nuclei. It is concerned in the more discriminative aspects of sensation, such as the qualities of shape, roughness, size and texture, and also in general awareness of the contralateral body image and the location of its parts. A lesion here may cause an inability to identify familiar objects manually (tactile

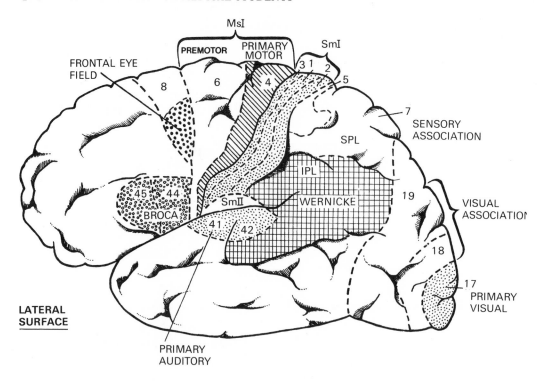

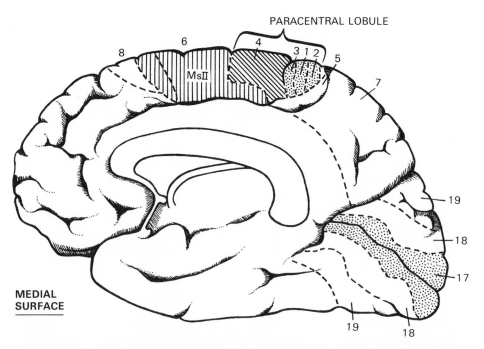

Fig. 12.8 The cerebral cortex showing the functional and cytoarchitectural (Brodmann) areas (1–45). **SPL**, superior parietal lobule: **IPL**, inferior parietal lobule; **Ms I**, precentral somatomotor; **Ms II**, supplementary somatomotor; **Sm I**, primary somatosensory; **Sm II**, supplementary somatosensory.

agnosia). An afflicted individual may appear unaware of the side of the body opposite to the lesion, neglecting to wash or shave it.

The *inferior parietal lobule* functions with the posterosuperior part of the temporal lobe; the combined region is *Wernicke's area* and is concerned with the interpretation of language through visual and auditory input. Sensory and motor 'speech areas' exist only in one hemisphere, the left in right-handed individuals, and this is the 'dominant hemisphere'. Damage results in word-blindness, *alexia*, and an inability to copy, *agraphia*, both being forms of *sensory aphasia*, the inability to understand written and spoken language.

Occipital lobe

The *primary visual area* (Brodmann area 17) is in the walls and floor of the posterior part of the calcarine sulcus, sometimes extending round the occipital pole to the lateral surface. Input is from the lateral geniculate body via the geniculocalcarine tract in the optic radiation. Histological features of the striate cortex have been described above; its columnar organization is described in Chapter 11. The left visual field projects to the right visual cortex; the superior retinal quadrants (lower visual field) project to the upper wall of the calcarine sulcus, inferior quadrants (upper field) to the lower; the macula has extensive representation, occupying approximately the posterior third of the primary visual area.

The *visual association area* (Brodmann areas 18, 19) occupies most of the remaining occipital cortex. It receives input from Brodmann area 17 and has reciprocal connexions with the pulvinar (in the cat and the monkey there is some input from the lateral geniculate body). It is concerned with the further abstraction and analysis of visual information; some neurons are specialized for the perception of colour. In general it relates present to past visual experience: a lesion may affect visual recognition. As a centre for automatic scanning, its solitary cells (of Meynert) form a corticocollicular connexion which, via the superior colliculus, co-ordinates involuntary eye movements, as in following moving objects. Unilateral stimulation produces contralateral conjugate deviation of the eyes. This area is linked with a 'frontal eye field' which activates voluntary scanning (*see* control of eye movements).

Temporal lobe

The human temporal neocortex is highly evolved; during development, part of it is submerged in the lateral fissure: two *transverse temporal gyri* (of Heschl) form its floor, bounded medially by the *insula*. The inferomedial margin, derived from the more primitive allocortex, is in-rolled as the *hippocampal formation* in the floor of the lateral ventricle's inferior horn. The temporal lobe has diverse functions such as linguistic interpretation, auditory, vestibular and visceral functions; its anterior pole ('psychical cortex') and hippocampal formation are involved in memory and behaviour. Connexions with the limbic system extend the functions of the temporal lobe beyond its physical boundaries.

The *primary auditory area* (Brodmann areas 41, 42) is mostly in the two transverse temporal gyri (of Heschl), extending slightly to the outer surface of the superior temporal gyrus. Area 41 is heterotypical granular cortex; area 42 is homotypical and is mainly an auditory association area. Input from the medial geniculate body is via the auditory radiation, which also includes some efferent fibres *to* the body and the inferior colliculus, concerned with selectivity and neural sharpening. A tonotopic representation has been described, with low frequencies anteriorly and high frequencies posteriorly in the area. Since auditory input is bilateral, a unilateral cortical lesion causes some deafness in both ears; if the damaged area is in the dominant hemisphere, comprehension of language is affected. The *auditory association area* is posteroinferior to the primary cortex and is linked with the inferior parietal lobule of the dominant hemisphere as Wernicke's area; it is essential to linguistic comprehension.

Vestibular representation is uncertain, but probably adjoins the 'face area' of Sm I. The *insula*, submerged in the lateral fissure, is surrounded by a circular sulcus and overlapped by the frontal, parietal and temporal *opercula*; its connexions are uncertain; stimulation in man evokes visceromotor and sensory effects such as nausea, salivation, gastrointestinal movements and alterations in blood pressure.

The *anterior part of the temporal lobe* ('psychical cortex') is described in Chapter 10 with the Klüver-Bucy syndrome and abnormal behavioural sequelae to bilateral ablation of this and the hippocampal formations. Stimulation may evoke visual or auditory memories, sometimes accompanied by fear; tumours may cause visual or auditory hallucinations. Lesions of the uncus may be associated with olfactory and gustatory hallucinations known as 'uncinate fits'.

Frontal lobe

The frontal cortex is divisible into a somatomotor *precentral region*, anterior to the central sulcus, and a larger *prefrontal association cortex*.

The precentral region or *first somatomotor area*, Ms I, includes the *precentral gyrus* (Brodmann area 4) and the *premotor area* (Brodmann area 6); the latter occupies the posterior parts of superior, middle and inferior frontal gyri. Both are agranular heterotypical cortex with numerous pyramidal neurons, but they differ physiologically; it is hence customary to designate them respectively 'primary motor' and 'premotor'. The corpus striatum and cerebellum project to Ms I via the ventral anterior and ventral lateral thalamic nuclei. The area is also influenced via non-specific thalamic afferents, by visual, acoustic and general sensory input; through numerous links with other cortical regions a great deal of interacting information underlies all 'executive' responses. Though it is the major source of corticospinal and corticobulbar fibres, some of these originate in the somatosensory areas posterior to the central sulcus. The frontal eye field and motor speech area are immediately anterior to the premotor area.

The *primary motor area* (Brodmann area 4) is in the anterior wall of the central sulcus and adjacent precentral gyrus, extending to the anterior part of the paracentral lobule on the medial surface, an area wider superiorly than inferiorly (*Fig.* 12.8). Giant pyramidal cells (of Betz), up to 120 μm in diameter, are most numerous in its superomedial part: about 3% of the pyramidal fibres originate in them, the majority being derived from smaller pyramidal neurons. Approximately 40% of pyramidal fibres (corticospinal and corticobulbar) come from Brodmann area 4, 20% from the postcentral gyrus and the remainder from the premotor area and parietal association cortex. Cortical somatotopic representation in Brodmann area 4 is in the form of an inverted homunculus (*Fig.* 12.9) in which the size of bodily regions is related to motor skill rather than to muscle bulk: thus the face, tongue, larynx and hand are disproportionately large, the trunk and lower extremities small. Appropriate electrical stimulation usually produces simple contraction of contralateral muscle groups. Skilled movements require intricate synaptic interactions which cannot be experimentally evoked. Bilateral movements occur in the masticatory, laryngeal, pharyngeal, upper facial and extra-ocular muscles. There are also 'centres' for the control of micturition and defaecation in the superomedial parts of the frontal lobes. Ablation of Brodmann area 4 in primates intitially results in flaccid paralysis, then partial recovery with impairment of skill, particularly in fine digital movements and in the distal limb muscles. Excessive stimulation produces 'pattern convulsions' similar to Jacksonian epilepsy, spreading from a focus in orderly progression throughout the body.

The *premotor area* (Brodmann area 6) is anterior to the primary motor area, and like the latter is wider superiorly than inferiorly and extends onto the medial surface. The cortical origins of the extrapyramidal fibres (corticostriate, corticorubral, cortico-olivary, corticoreticular, corticonigral) are diffuse, but are particularly related to this

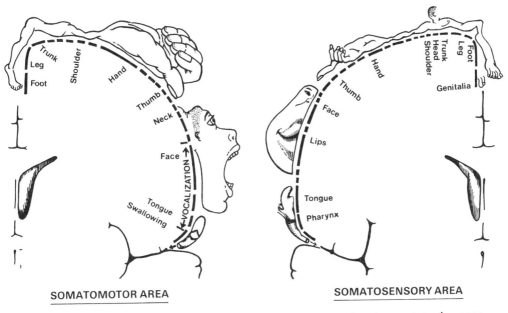

SOMATOMOTOR AREA

SOMATOSENSORY AREA

Fig. 12.9 Motor and sensory homunculi showing proportional somatotopic representation in the cortex. (After Penfield W. and Rasmussen T. (1950) *The Cerebral Cortex of Man.* London, Macmillan.)

area. To produce movements, stronger stimulation is required than in Brodmann area 4 and the movement patterns are more generalized and often postural, for example rotation of the head, eyes and trunk, flexion or extension of the limbs.

The *supplementary motor area*, Ms II, is on the medial surface of the frontal lobe (Brodmann areas 6, part of 8), anterior to, and blending with, the paracentral lobule. In monkeys the body is represented horizontally, with the head anterior; human somatotopic representation is not known. The area's significance is not clear: stimulation produces bilateral co-ordinated postural movements: unilateral ablation in man produces no permanent functional loss.

The *frontal eye field*, situated caudally in the middle frontal gyrus, occupies the inferolateral part of Brodmann area 8 and includes parts of the adjoining areas 6 and 9. Stimulation causes contralateral conjugate ocular deviation. It is said to be a 'centre for voluntary scanning', in consciously-directed movements, as in searching visual fields for particular features.

The *motor speech area of Broca* (Brodmann areas 44, 45) is situated caudally in the inferior frontal gyrus of the dominant hemisphere, on the left side in right-handed individuals, the same side as Wernicke's area. Dominance of one hemisphere is genetically determined; right- or left-handedness may be influenced by educational and other factors. Lesions in this area result in *motor aphasia*: although language is understood, it cannot be expressed in speech or writing.

The *prefrontal area* includes those parts of the frontal lobe not yet described. It has reciprocal connexions with dorsal medial and anterior thalamic nuclei through the anterior thalamic radiation, and with the hypothalamus and corpus striatum; frontopontine fibres project to the cerebellum via the nuclei pontis. Association fibres connect with the parietal, occipital and temporal lobes. Commissural fibres of the forceps minor and the genu of the corpus callosum unite corresponding parts of the frontal cortices. Until the discovery of specific anti-depressant drugs, prefrontal leucotomy was sometimes performed, bilaterally severing the thalamic connexions of the orbito-frontal cortex. The post-operative sequelae illustrate the functions of this area, for example relieved depression, altered affective tone and reduced emotional content of pain. Extensive bilateral frontal lobe injuries have a detrimental effect not only on emotional balance, but on behaviour and intellect, resulting in a profound change of personality. The prefrontal cortex is concerned with depth of emotion, with social, moral and ethical awareness, and with the ability to concentrate, to elaborate ideas and to solve problems; it is also concerned with planning, foresight, judgement, the correlation and evaluation of information and the choice of appropriate responses.

GENERAL CONSIDERATIONS

Cerebral dominance

In manual dexterity and linguistic skill the left hemisphere is genetically dominant in right-handed individuals; the human brain appears unique in this respect. Left-handedness is a less definite phenomenon and is not necessarily related to cerebral dominance. Imperfectly developed dominance may be associated with difficulties in reading, writing, drawing and spatial analysis. Whereas the dominant hemisphere is concerned with language and mathematical and analytical functions, spatial and pictorial concepts appear to be processed more in the non-dominant hemisphere. The myelination and function of the corpus callosum are incomplete until two or three years after birth, during which time both hemispheres process linguistic information. Young children sustaining damage to a dominant left hemisphere can become skillfully left-handed and can learn to speak, read and write, utilizing the early neuronal plasticity which is lost as age progresses. (For a general view of neuronal plasticity *see* Cotman, 1978).

Sleep

Sleep *was* regarded as a purely passive state, a nocturnal depression of the reticular activating system. It is *now* known to be an active and complex process with two contrasting and alternating intrinsic rhythms, separately identifiable by encephalography and controlled from brainstem centres by specific neurotransmitters.

Slow wave sleep is characterized by synchronized high voltage, low frequency, encephalographic waves. Most muscles relax, but postural adjustments occur. There is parasympathetic dominance: the heart rate and blood pressure decrease, respiration is slow and regular and gastrointestinal movements are increased.

Paradoxical sleep, occuring at intervals during the night, is associated with ocular movements, and is named 'paradoxical' because encephalography shows desynchronized, low voltage, fast waves, like those seen in the waking state. Sympathetic activity evokes a raised heart rate and blood pressure, respiration is rapid and irregular and gastrointestinal movements are decreased. Muscle tone is depressed, apart from characteristic bursts of rapid eye movements; hence the alternative name 'REM sleep'. The ocular movements are triggered by phasic electrical activity in the pontine reticular formation, lateral geniculate bodies and occipital cortex, known as ponto-geniculo-occipital (PGO) spikes; these are probably initiated by ascending impulses from the medial and inferior vestibular nuclei.

The *pontine raphé nuclei* contain serotonin (5–HT) and are involved in slow wave sleep; those in the caudal pons act as a priming mechanism for paradoxical sleep. Damage to the nuclei of the raphé is said to produce total insomnia. The *locus caeruleus*, near the periaqueductal grey matter, contains noradrenaline (norepinephrine) and is active in paradoxical sleep; there is also evidence that acetylcholine is involved in this process. These complex interrelationships are incompletely understood.

Memory

It is necessary to distinguish between input, storage and retrieval of information. The hippocampal formations have a particular role in memory input; lesions of the limbic system may impair this. The anterior parts of the temporal lobe appear to be concerned not only with input but also with storage: electrical stimulation may result in recall of previous experience. Learning requires a storage of information. Experimental ablation of any area of the cortex slows the rate of learning in proportion to the area lost; certain regions have additional specific contributions, for example the visual and auditory regions. Even mild but diffuse cortical compression, as by chronic subdural haematoma, leads to impaired learning and memory.

The extent of dendritic fields and complexity of intracortical circuits increase in response to sustained and varied input; conversely, inactivity causes thinning of the cortex. Blindness leads to atrophy of the visual cortex, and neonatal monocular deprivation permanently affects ocular dominance (*see* p. 185). The plasticity of the central nervous system is most active in youth. 'Old dogs cannot learn new tricks', but experience and the resultant ability to evaluate increases with age. Old age generally entails defective memory for recent events, recall of distant events being unaffected; this is a normal phenomenon, differing from 'senile dementia', in which there is generalized cerebral atrophy, often with a profound change in personality. The reverberating circuits which encode short-term memory may also be disrupted by deep anaesthesia or trauma, leaving long-term memory unaffected; this implies a more permanent physical change for the latter, though its nature remains obscure. The prefrontal cortex is necessary for the motivation and concentration required in complex learning processes.

APPLIED ANATOMY

Functional correlations of cortical areas have been mentioned in this chapter. Damage to these may result from a cerebrovascular accident (CVA), such as haemorrhage, thrombosis or embolism, or from cerebral tumours, other forms of intracranial compression, or in head injuries (*see* also p. 228). Major localizing symptoms are summarized:

Motor cortex. Damage to the *precentral area* produces spastic paralysis of the contralateral limbs; normally extrapyramidal fibres from this area inhibit muscle tone. If one *frontal eye field* is affected, the eyes 'look to the side of the lesion'. Destruction of the *motor speech area* results in expressive (motor) aphasia or an inability to speak, linguistic comprehension being unaffected.

An unusual example of neuronal plasticity is demonstrated in a middle-aged patient who, *as a young child,* had the right cerebral hemisphere removed because of severe epilepsy; although he has little useful movement of the left hand, he can walk almost normally. In such cases, areas of the *developing* central nervous system may assume some of the functions of missing components; this capacity is lost after early childhood.

Sensory cortex. Lesions of the *primary somatosensory area* result in contralateral loss of sensory discrimination, although crude awareness, particularly of nociceptive stimuli, is retained at thalamic level. Dysfunction of the *somatosensory association areas* leads to tactile agnosia, that is inability to appreciate three-dimensional shape (astereognosis), size, weight or texture when identifying familiar objects by touch; there is also a lack of awareness of the body's contralateral side. The non-dominant parietal lobe has a more general capacity for pictorial and spatial analysis; lesions may result in an inability to arrange the sequential components of complex movements, a form of apraxia. Sensory aphasia, the inability to recognize spoken or written words, follows damage to *Wernicke's area* in the dominant hemisphere. Lesions of the *primary visual area* cause contralateral visual field loss proportional to the extent of the damage. Defects of the *visual association areas* impair visual recognition. A lesion in the lateral fissure may affect the *primary auditory area* causing partial bilateral deafness, the vestibular area causing vertigo, and the insula causing visceral effects such as nausea, salivation and altered blood pressure. The personality may be severely affected by bilateral damage to the *prefrontal cortex* or the *temporal lobes*.

Fetal neurons may survive when implanted experimentally into senile rat brains; cells containing acetylcholine appear to improve memory, dopamine cells improve balance.

Chapter 13

Meninges and cerebrospinal fluid

Three continuous membranes or *meninges*, the dura mater, arachnoid mater and pia mater, surround the brain and spinal cord. Their intracranial arrangement differs from that in the vertebral canal and will be described separately.

INTRACRANIAL MENINGES

Dura mater

This is often regarded as bilaminar, with an external *endosteal layer* of periosteum, continuous through the cranial foramina and sutures with the pericranium, and an internal *meningeal layer*, a strong fibrous membrane continuous with the vertebral dura mater at the foramen magnum. The meningeal dura mater and endosteum are adherent except where *dural venous sinuses* intervene. Meningeal dura mater ensheathes the cranial nerves in their osseous foramina, fusing externally with their epineurium; the sheaths of the optic nerves fuse with the ocular sclera.

The meningeal dura mater is infolded as septa between parts of the brain (*Fig.* 13.1). The sickle-shaped median *falx cerebri*, between the cerebral hemispheres, is narrow anteriorly where it is attached to the ethmoid crista galli and wider posteriorly where it joins the horizontal tentorium cerebelli. Its upper convex margin, attached to endosteum parasagittally as far as the internal occipital protruberance, encloses a *superior sagittal sinus*; its unattached lower concave edge contains an *inferior sagittal sinus*. The *straight sinus*, formed by the junction of the inferior sagittal sinus and the great cerebral vein, runs in the attachment of the falx cerebri to the tentorium cerebelli.

The *tentorium cerebelli*, roofing the posterior cranial fossa, is between the cerebellum and the cerebral occipital lobes. Its anterior free edge borders the *tentorial incisure*, in which lies the midbrain. Its peripheral border is attached posteriorly to the margins of the occipital grooves for the *transverse sinuses*, bilaterally to the superior edges of the petrous temporal bones (where it encloses the *superior petrosal sinuses*) and anteriorly to the posterior clinoid processes of the sphenoid bone. The free edge extends forwards to the anterior clinoid processes, crossing the attached border; here the oculomotor and trochlear nerves pierce the meningeal dura mater to enter the lateral wall of the *cavernous sinus* on each side. Near the apices of the petrous temporal bones, the

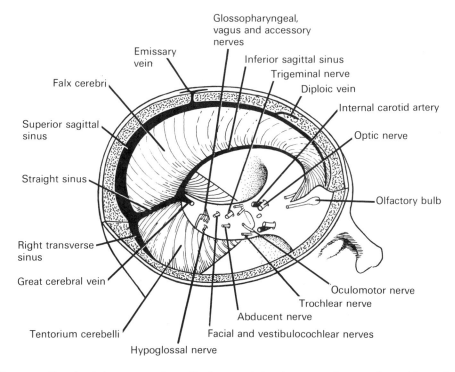

Fig. 13.1 Cerebral dura mater, its reflexions and dural venous sinuses viewed from the superolateral aspect, the brain having been removed.

meningeal dura mater is evaginated under each superior petrosal sinus as a *cavum trigeminale*, partially enclosing the trigeminal ganglion.

The smaller *falx cerebelli* extends down from the tentorium cerebelli in the posterior cerebellar notch; at its attachment to the internal occipital crest it encloses an *occipital sinus*. The *diaphragma sellae* roofs the sella turcica, perforated by the pituitary infundibulum.

The *dural arterial supply* is from numerous rami of the internal carotid, ascending pharyngeal, maxillary, occipital and vertebral arteries. The *middle meningeal artery*, branching from the maxillary artery, traverses the foramen spinosum to lie between the endosteal and meningeal dura mater. Its anterior and posterior branches groove and supply bones of the cranial vault with meningeal veins between the arteries and bone. The anterior (frontal) branch crosses the pterion, the posterior (parietal) ascends backwards towards the lambda. A fracture of the thin squamous temporal bone may cause a 'middle meningeal haemorrhage' from the artery or vein, producing an *extra-dural haematoma*. The nerve supply to the supratentorial dura is trigeminal, while the infratentorial supply is from the vagus and the upper three cervical nerves.

Dural venous sinuses (*Figs.* 13.1, 13.2, 6.15)

The venous sinuses, sited between the meningeal and endosteal layers of dura mater, are lined by endothelium, have no valves, and drain to the internal jugular veins. They have

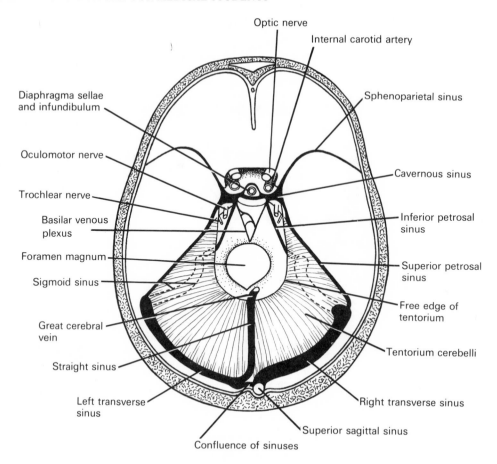

Fig. 13.2 Superior aspect of the tentorium cerebelli with the venous sinuses exposed.

cerebral, diploic and some meningeal tributaries and, through skull foramina, communicate via valveless emissary veins with extracranial vessels.

The *superior sagittal sinus*, in the attached border of the falx cerebri, extends from the foramen caecum (where it may communicate with nasal veins) to the internal occipital protruberance, continuing there usually into the right transverse sinus at the *confluence of the sinuses*. Here it communicates with the left transverse, occipital and straight sinuses. Large clusters of *arachnoid villi*, concerned in the absorption of cerebrospinal fluid, form *arachnoid granulations* projecting into the *venous lacunae* of the superior sagittal sinus (*Fig.* 13.3). As these granulations enlarge with age they create parasagittal depressions in the inner surface of the cranial vault. *Superior cerebral veins* ascend slightly anteriorly to the superior sagittal sinus and its lacunae; they thus traverse the subdural space (between dura and arachnoid): traumatic posterior displacement of the brain may tear these veins, causing *subdural haemorrhage*.

The *inferior sagittal sinus*, in the lower border of the falx cerebri, communicates with the medial cerebral veins and, joined by the *great cerebral vein*, forms the *straight sinus* at the junction of the falx cerebri and tentorium cerebelli. At the confluence of the sinuses the straight sinus usually turns into the left transverse sinus. The paired *transverse sinuses*, in the attached margin of the tentorium cerebelli, groove the occipital bone; they become *sigmoid sinuses* on the internal aspects of the mastoid temporal bones, continuing as the internal jugular veins posteriorly in the jugular foramina. Each transverse sinus receives the superior petrosal sinus and the inferior cerebral and cerebellar veins. The *occipital sinus*, in the falx cerebelli, extends from the confluence of the sinuses to the foramen magnum, where it communicates with the vertebral venous plexus.

Cavernous sinuses (*Fig.* 6.15) flank the sphenoid's body from the superior orbital fissures to the apices of the petrous temporal bones, and are so named because of their internal trabeculation. Each is traversed by an internal carotid artery, its sympathetic plexus and an abducent nerve, covered by endothelium. In the lateral wall of each sinus, between the endothelium and the meningeal dura mater, are the oculomotor and trochlear nerves and the ophthalmic and maxillary trigeminal branches. The two sinuses are connected by veins in the diaphragma sellae; anteriorly they communicate with *ophthalmic veins*, and hence with the facial vein; facial infection may thus spread to the cavernous sinuses, a potentially fatal event prior to the discovery of antibiotics. Each sinus receives a *superficial middle cerebral vein* and a *sphenoparietal sinus*, a small channel under the lesser wing of the sphenoid bone. A *basilar venous plexus* crosses the clivus to the foramen magnum, communicating there with the vertebral veins. Posteriorly each cavernous sinus drains via a *superior petrosal sinus* to the transverse sinus, and via an *inferior petrosal sinus* through the jugular foramen to the internal jugular's bulb. A number of *emissary veins* connect each cavernous sinus with the internal jugular vein, pterygoid and pharyngeal plexuses, through the foramina ovale, spinosum, lacerum and jugulare.

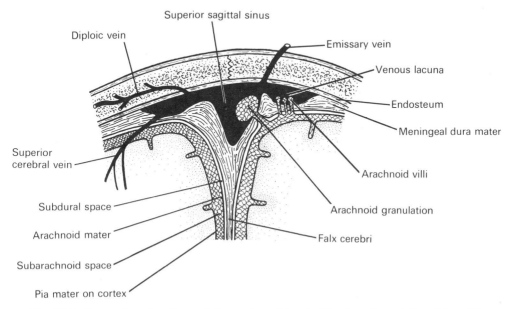

Fig. 13.3 Coronal section through the vertex of the skull to show the relationships of the superior sagittal sinus and the meninges.

Arachnoid mater and pia mater

Between the meningeal dura mater and the arachnoid mater a cleavage plane, the *subdural space*, is traversed only by cerebral veins en route to the dural venous sinuses. In contrast, the *subarachnoid space*, between the arachnoid mater and the pia mater, contains a web of trabeculae (arachnoid = spidery), cerebrospinal fluid, cerebral arteries and veins. The *pia mater* is vascular and closely bound to the cortical surfaces of gyri and sulci by a *glial membrane*, surrounding blood vessels as they enter the cortex to form *perivascular spaces*, which are shallow extensions of the subarachnoid space (*Fig.* 13.4). The *arachnoid mater* is a delicate, impermeable, avascular membrane; unlike the pia mater, it bridges sulci and other surface irregularities. The width of the subarachnoid space is therefore variable, narrow over gyri, wider over sulci and cerebral fissures and wider still at the cerebral base, where it forms subarachnoid cisterns (*Fig.* 13.5). Into the largest, the *cerebellomedullary cistern* (cistern magna), between the cerebellum and medulla, cerebrospinal fluid escapes from the fourth ventricle via the median and lateral apertures (of Magendie and Luschka). Other cisterns are the *pontine, interpeduncular, chiasmatic* and *superior*. The superior cistern, together with the subarachnoid spaces lateral to the midbrain, is termed the *cisterna ambiens* by clinicians: it contains the great cerebral vein and the posterior cerebral and superior cerebellar arteries. (The cisterns and ventricles can be examined radiographically, *see* Applied Anatomy).

The subarachnoid space surrounds each cranial nerve for a short distance at its foramen. Around the optic nerves the space reaches the sclera; the central retinal artery

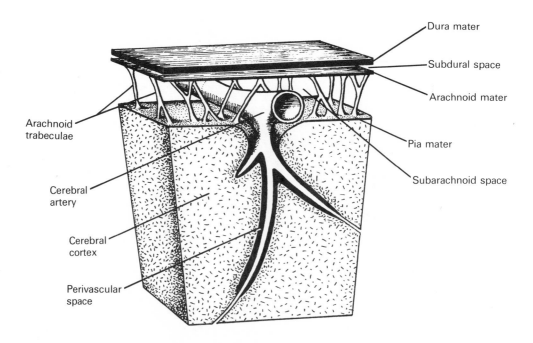

Fig. 13.4 A section through the cerebral meninges, subarachnoid and perivascular spaces.

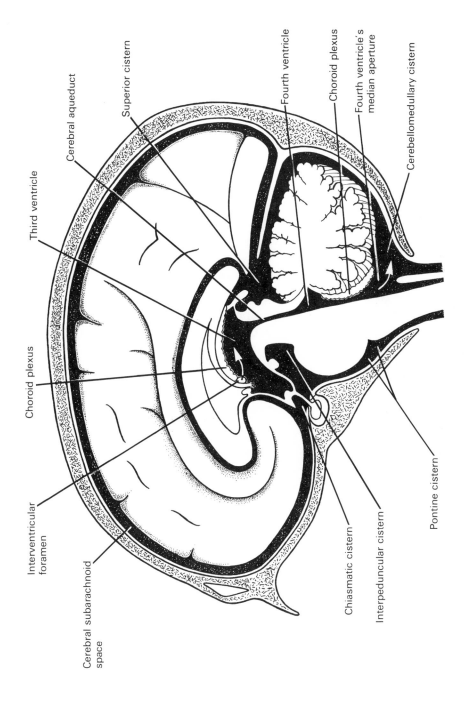

Cerebral aqueduct

Superior cistern

Third ventricle

Choroid plexus

Interventricular foramen

Cerebral subarachnoid space

Chiasmatic cistern

Interpeduncular cistern

Pontine cistern

Fourth ventricle

Choroid plexus

Fourth ventricle's median aperture

Cerebellomedullary cistern

Fig. 13.5 Median sagittal section to show the subarachnoid cisterns. Arrows in the interventricular foramen and in the median aperture of the fourth ventricle indicate the circulation of cerebrospinal fluid.

and vein cross it, and raised cerebrospinal fluid pressure may compress the vein, causing oedema of the optic disc or *papilloedema*.

Ventricular choroid plexuses develop where the pia mater and ependyma are in contact (*see* below, cerebrospinal fluid).

SPINAL MENINGES

The *spinal dura mater*, continuous with the intracranial dura mater, is attached to the edge of the foramen magnum, the bodies of the second and third cervical vertebrae and the posterior longitudinal vertebral ligament. *Arachnoid mater* adheres to its internal aspect, and both meninges extend to second sacral vertebral level, where the dura mater blends with the filum terminale. The dura mater and arachnoid mater are evaginated by the spinal nerve roots, fusing with the epineurium just beyond the dorsal root ganglia (*Fig.* 4.2). The *extradural (epidural) space* is extensive, containing a valveless vertebral venous plexus, arteries, fat and lymphatics. Local anaesthetics may be injected into it, a procedure termed 'epidural anaesthesia'. The *pia mater* closely invests the spinal cord and roots, thickened along its anterior sulcus as a *linea splendens* and drawn out as a bilateral *denticulate ligament* with twenty-one 'teeth' attached to the arachnoid mater and dura mater. The *subarachnoid space* is not trabecular. Distal to the spinal cord, the *lumbar cistern* extends from the second lumbar to the second sacral vertebrae and contains the cauda equina (lumbosacral nerve roots) and filum terminale. A needle may be inserted safely into the cistern in the third or fourth lumbar interspinous spaces; if strictly median this should not touch the nerve roots.

CEREBROSPINAL FLUID

Cerebrospinal fluid (CSF) is secreted by the choroid plexuses in all the ventricles, but mostly in the lateral ventricles, whose plexuses are the largest. Where the pia mater and its vessels contact the ependyma, the two form a double membrane, the *tela choroidea*, with vascular fringes (*see* development, Chapter 1). The arrangement of the choroid plexuses in the lateral and third ventricles is shown in *Figs*. 13.6 and 13.7. A tela choroidea roofs the third ventricle, plexuses in its margins invaginating the medial wall of each lateral ventricle through a *choroid fissure*. Each fissure extends posteriorly from an interventricular foramen; in the lateral ventricle's body it is bounded superiorly by the fornix, inferiorly by the thalamus; in its inferior horn it is between the stria terminalis above and the fimbria below. Posteriorly the tela is in the *transverse fissure* between the splenium above and the junction of the tectum and the third ventricle's roof below; it is interposed between the telencephalon and diencephalon during development.

A choroid plexus has a convoluted surface, covered by a single layer of cuboidal epithelium whose cells have apical microvilli and a basement membrane (*Fig.* 13.8).

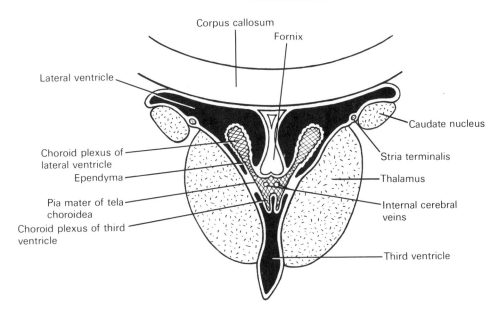

Fig. 13.6 Coronal section posterior to the interventricular foramen showing the choroid plexuses of the third and lateral ventricles.

Epithelial tight junctions form a *blood/CSF barrier*. The presence of numerous mitochondria indicates that secretion of CSF is at least partly an active metabolic process. The subjacent stroma contains many capillaries, some fenestrated, supplied by the anterior and posterior choroidal branches of the internal carotid and posterior cerebral arteries respectively. Approximately 30% of CSF by volume is derived from neural metabolism and filtration from non-choroidal capillaries.

A brain of 1500 g weighs only 50 g when submerged in CSF. This protects the brain's semi-solid structure and moderates the effects of sudden displacement, resisting concussion. Cerebrospinal fluid provides the special environment essential for neural tissue: there is no barrier to diffusion between them. It has a much lower protein content than blood plasma (6.5 g protein/100 g plasma; 0.025 g protein/100 g CSF); the glucose content is about half that of blood, the chloride content slightly more in CSF. Normally clear and colourless, with a specific gravity of 1.003–1.008, it has less than 5 lymphocytes/mm^3. In bacterial meningitis the fluid is cloudy, with raised protein content and a vastly increased number of cells. Analysis of it has diagnostic value in many central nervous diseases.

Cerebrospinal fluid volume averages 140 ml, of which 23 ml is intraventricular. From the lateral to the third ventricle, via the cerebral aqueduct to the fourth ventricle and thence via the median and lateral apertures to the subarachnoid space, about 500 ml is passed daily. Absorption into the venous sinuses is through the arachnoid villi, which act as valves, opened when the CSF pressure exceeds the venous pressure. There is also some absorption via small spinal veins into the vertebral venous system.

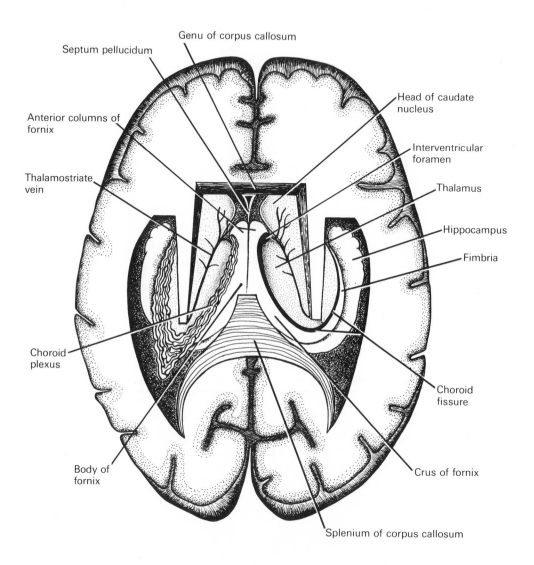

Fig. 13.7 A dissection of the lateral ventricles viewed from the superior aspect: on the right side the choroid plexus has been removed to reveal the choroid fissure.

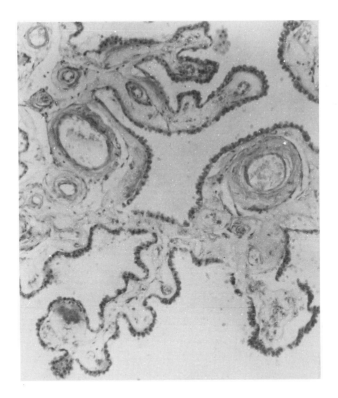

Fig. 13.8 A section of choroid plexus. Note the large capillaries and convoluted epithelium. (Haematoxylin and eosin, × 125.)

The pressure CSF, 80–180 ml of saline, is measured with the patient horizontal, a needle in the lumbar cistern connected to a manometer. The pressure is increased by coughing, straining or sitting up. It is also raised by manual compression of the internal jugular veins, indicating normal communication between the cerebral and spinal subarachnoid spaces (Queckenstedt's sign).

BLOOD/BRAIN BARRIER

Selective filtration is necessary to provide the particular environment required by the central nervous system. The blood/brain and blood/CSF barriers and the free diffusion between brain and CSF are illustrated diagrammatically:

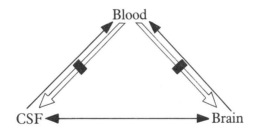

A blood/CSF barrier was noted above in description of choroid plexuses.

Intravenous vital dyes stain most tissues except the brain. The blood/brain barrier is due largely to a continuous capillary lining of endothelial cells with tight junctions. In addition, 85% of the capillary basement membrane is covered by the 'end feet' of astrocytes (*Fig.* 2.6), a selective nutritive path to neurons. Intravascular chemicals may enter the brain either because they are lipid-soluble, or by active transport mechanisms (carrier mediation) in the endothelium and the glia, which contain enzymes controlling the transport of amines, amino acids and sugars. Thus, dopamine cannot pass but L–dopa can; having entered the endothelium it is converted there to dopamine. In Parkinson's disease there is dopamine deficiency, alleviated by the administration of L–dopa.

Some diseases cause a 'breakdown' of the blood/brain barrier. Normally penicillin cannot enter the central nervous system: it has low lipid solubility, is bound to plasma albumin, and the choroid plexus transports it from the CSF to the blood. However, in bacterial meningitis, encephalitis and uraemia, penicillin crosses the barrier. There may also be a local breakdown in brain tumours; radioactive-labelled albumin then enters the tumour tissue selectively, facilitating diagnosis and localization.

Certain small cerebral regions with secretary functions have fenestrated capillaries; these include the pineal gland, neurohypophysis and hypothalamic median eminence.

APPLIED ANATOMY

The cranium contains the brain, blood and CSF, an increase in the volume of any one of which results in the decrease of another. Compensation is possible within physiological limits; sneezing or straining cause transient venous congestion, but some CSF may be displaced through the foramen magnum.

In *hydrocephalus* the CSF is increased in volume and, before the fusion of the cranial sutures, the skull may greatly enlarge. In *internal hydrocephalus* the ventricular system is obstructed, commonly at the fourth ventricle's foramina, due to basal meningitis, but sometimes due to congenital stenosis of the aqueduct. In *communicating hydrocephalus* the obstruction is outside the brain, for example adhesions between the midbrain and the tentorial incisure, or blockage of arachnoid granulations after meningitis. The brain is compressed and the cortex atrophies. In *senile dementia*, cerebral atrophy is accompanied by a compensatory enlargement of the subarachnoid space and ventricles.

Cerebral oedema, due to an impaired blood/brain barrier, may follow head injury, meningitis, cerebral anoxia, uraemia and other toxic conditions, leading to coma.

Raised intracranial pressure causes papilloedema, slow pulse, raised blood pressure and impaired consciousness. *Radiological investigations* include the injection of radio-opaque fluid into the internal carotid or vertebral arteries (cerebral *angiography*, *Fig.* 14.5), injection of air into the ventricles (*ventriculography*, *Fig.* 13.9) or into the lumbar cistern (*encephalography*). These are now largely replaced by *computerized tomography* (CT scan, *Fig.* 13.10), a radiological technique producing serial cross-sections of the cranial contents.

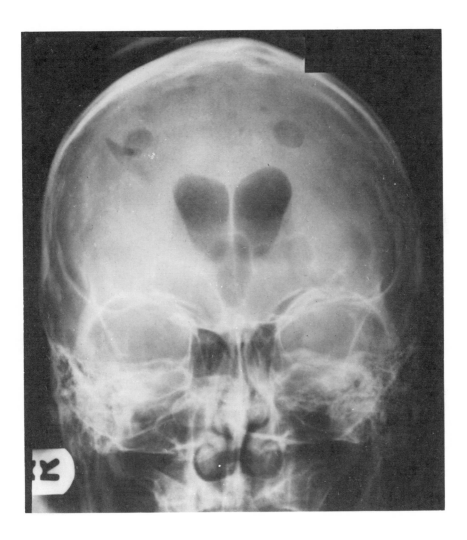

Fig. 13.9 A ventriculogram: air has been injected into the lateral ventricles through holes in the skull. Note the midline septum pellucidum.

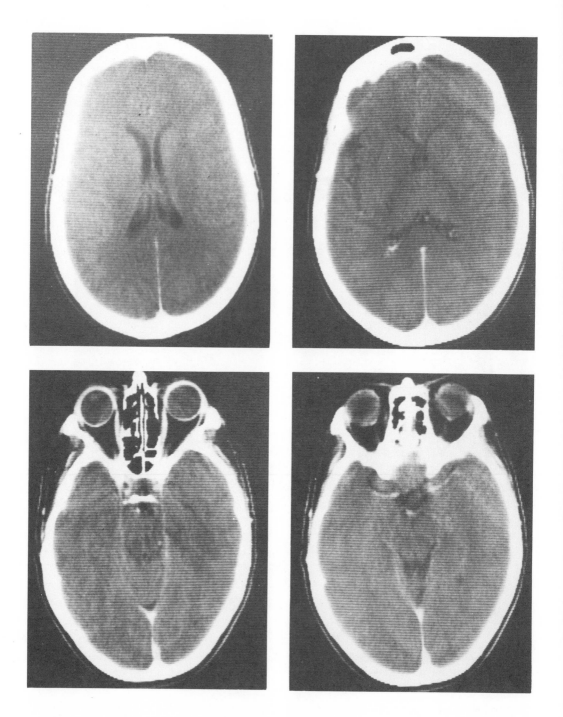

Fig. 13.10 Computerized tomography. These radiographic 'sections' of the brain are taken at an angle of 25° to the base line of the skull.

Chapter 14

Blood supply of the central nervous system

The brain requires active aerobic metabolism of glucose; if the arterial supply ceases for ten seconds, unconsciousness ensues, and after four minutes irreversible degeneration begins.

ARTERIES OF THE BRAIN

The brain is supplied by the paired internal carotid and vertebral arteries; all four anastomose on its inferior surface in the *circulus arteriosus* (of Willis) (*Fig.* 14.1), but the posterior communicating arteries are usually too slender to compensate for major obstruction. The cerebral and cerebellar arteries are in the subarachnoid space; their branches are either cortical or central, with little anastomosis between the superficial and deep areas supplied. Large *cortical branches* ramify in the pia mater; from them small rami enter the cortex and subcortical tissue. Surface anastomosis between the three major cerebral arteries is variable and usually limited; hence, if <u>one</u> is occluded, damage ensues. *Central branches* from the circulus arteriosus and adjacent parts of the three paired cerebral arteries supply the internal capsule, diencephalon and corpus striatum. These small but vital vessels form anteromedial, posteromedial, anterolateral and posterolateral groups (*Fig.* 14.1). The anterior and posterior choroidal branches, respectively from the internal carotid and posterior cerebral arteries, provide central as well as choroidal branches. Connexions between the individual central arteries is poor; hence their occlusion in the main cause of 'stroke'. The cerebral arteries and their rami have thinner walls than other vessels of similar diameter.

Each *internal carotid artery*, traversing its canal in the petrous temporal bone, enters the middle cranial fossa between the endosteum and the meningeal dura mater and turns forwards in the cavernous sinus. Its arched course thereafter is described as a 'carotid syphon' in angiograms (*Fig.* 14.5). Turning up medial to the anterior clinoid process, it pierces the meningeal dura mater and arachnoid mater, enters the subarachnoid space, runs back below the optic nerve and then lateral to the optic chiasma; there, subjacent to the anterior perforated substance, it divides into the *anterior and middle cerebral arteries*. Its intrapetrosal part gives off a *caroticotympanic* branch to the tympanic cavity, the intracavernous part supplies *hypophysial arteries* to the neuro-hypophysis and the median hypothalamic eminence; from the latter a portal system

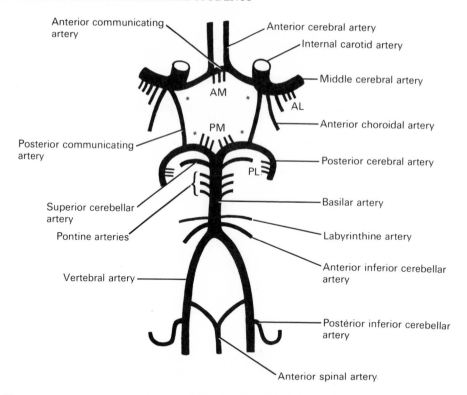

Fig. 14.1 Diagram of arteries at the base of the brain showing the circulus arteriosus*. The groups of central branches are anteromedial (**AM**), anterolateral (**AL**), postero-medial (**PM**) and posterolateral (**PL**).

extends to the adenohypophysis. Collateral branches within the subarachnoid space are the ophthalmic, posterior communicating and anterior choroidal arteries. The *ophthalmic artery* traverses the optic canal inferolateral to the optic nerve, supplies orbital structures, the frontal and ethmoidal air sinuses, the frontal area of scalp and the dorsum of nose. The *posterior communicating artery* arises near the terminal carotid bifurcation and runs posteriorly in the circulus arteriosus to join the posterior cerebral artery; usually slender, it is sometimes large and gives origin to the posterior cerebral artery. The *anterior choroidal artery* branches from the end of the internal carotid or from the commencement of the middle cerebral artery. Running posteriorly near the optic tract, it crosses the uncus to enter the choroidal plexus in the lateral ventricle's inferior horn. It also supplies the optic tract, lateral geniculate body, hippocampal formation, amygdaloid nucleus, globus pallidus, posterior limb and retrolentiform part of the internal capsule. Long and slender, it is prone to thrombosis.

Each *vertebral artery* ascends through the foramina transversaria of the upper six cervical vertebrae, curves behind the lateral mass of the atlas and pierces the atlanto-occipital membrane, dura mater and arachnoid mater to enter the posterior cranial fossa via the foramen magnum. The two vertebral arteries unite at the pontine lower border, forming the *basilar artery*, which ascends in the median pontine sulcus to bifurcate at the upper pontine border into two *posterior cerebral arteries*.

Cortical blood supply (*Fig.* 14.2, 14.3, 14.4, 14.5)

Each *anterior cerebral artery*, the smaller terminal carotid branch, runs anteromedially above the optic nerve towards the longitudinal fissure, united there to its fellow by a short *anterior communicating artery*. Both then arch over the callosal genu, coursing posteriorly as the *pericallosal arteries* on the corpus, each giving off a *callosomarginal branch* which follows the sulcus cinguli. The cortical supply is to the orbital surface of the frontal lobe, to the medial hemispheric surface as far back as the parieto-occipital sulcus, and to an adjacent strip of the dorsolateral surface. This includes the 'leg area' of the motor cortex. Thrombosis of this vessel is uncommon.

Each *middle cerebral artery*, the larger branch and main continuation of the internal carotid artery, courses through the lateral fissure to the insula, supplying cortical rami to most of the dorsolateral surface (except a narrow superior strip supplied by the anterior cerebral artery, and the occipital pole and inferior border supplied by the posterior cerebral artery). This distribution includes the motor and sensory areas adjoining the

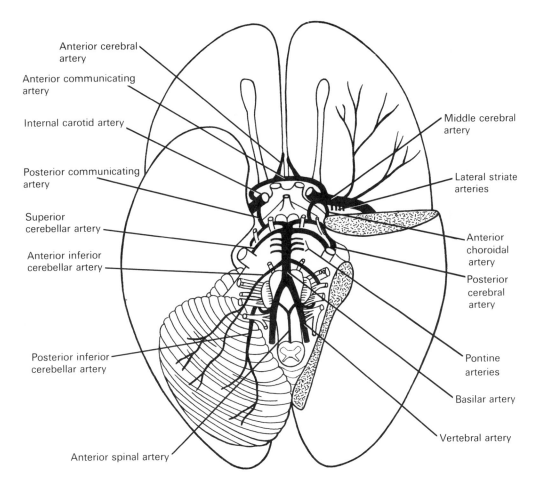

Fig. 14.2 Arteries at the base of the brain. The right cerebellar hemisphere and cerebral temporal lobe have been removed.

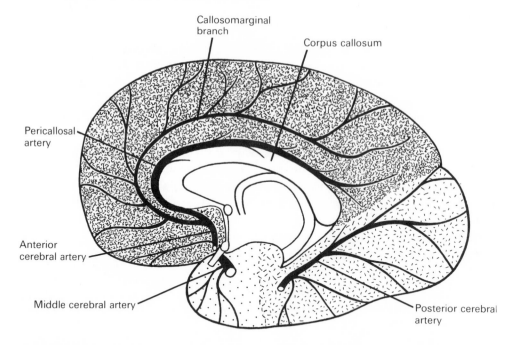

Fig. 14.3 The distribution of arteries on the medial surface of the right cerebral hemisphere.

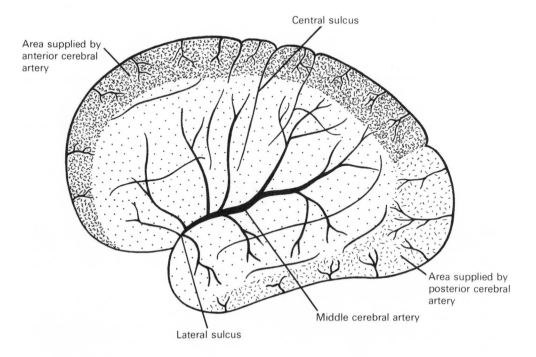

Fig. 14.4 The distribution of arteries on the lateral surface of the left cerebral hemisphere.

central sulcus (except the 'leg area') and, in the dominant hemisphere, the speech and language areas. Cerebral thrombosis most commonly affects this artery in its main, cortical or central branches.

The two *posterior cerebral arteries* are terminal rami for the basilar artery; both receive a posterior communicating vessel from the internal carotid artery and then arch posteriorly round the cerebral peduncles to the tentorial surface of the cerebrum. The cortical supply is to the occipital lobe (medial, inferior and part of the lateral surface) and to the inferior surface of the temporal lobe, including the parahippocampal gyrus and uncus. Vascular deprivation of the visual cortex causes blindness in the opposite visual field (contralateral homonymous hemianopia), often with 'macular sparing', the latter sometimes attributed to a branch of the middle cerebral artery reaching this area.

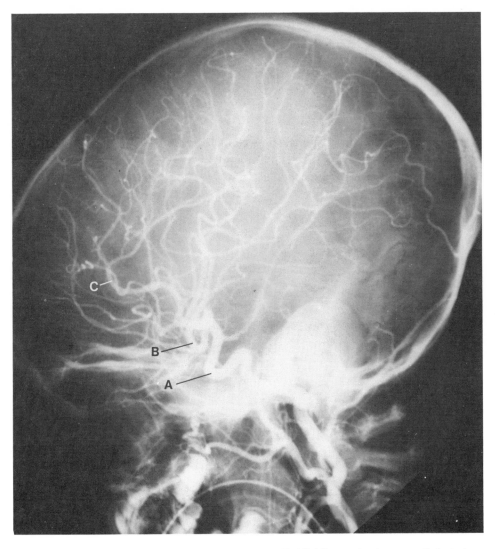

Fig. 14.5 Carotid angiogram. **A**, Carotid syphon; **B**, Middle cerebral artery; **C**, Anterior cerebral artery.

Central arteries

These small, deeply perforating branches are in four main groups (*Fig.* 14.1) but they occur elsewhere also.

1. The *anteromedial arteries*, arising from the anterior cerebral and anterior communicating arteries, enter via the anterior perforated substance to supply the anterior limb of the internal capsule, the head of the caudate nucleus, the putamen and the anterior hypothalamus. They include the *medial striate artery*.

2. The *anterolateral (lateral striate) arteries*, arising from the proximal part of the middle cerebral artery, pierce the anterior perforated substance to supply the anterior limb of the internal capsule and the caudate and lentiform nuclei. The largest ramus, and the most susceptible to rupture, is known as the 'artery of cerebral haemorrhage'. It is appropriate to include in this group the *anterior choroidal artery*, arising from the internal carotid, previously described; it supplies the posterior limb of the internal capsule.

3. The *posterolateral arteries*, arising from each posterior cerebral artery after it has curved round the cerebral peduncle, supply the peduncle and the posterior part of the thalamus, including the geniculate bodies.

4. The *posteromedial arteries*, from the proximal part of the posterior cerebral and posterior communicating arteries, supply the cerebral peduncle and enter the posterior perforated substance (between the peduncles), supplying the anterior part of the thalamus, the subthalamus and the central and posterior regions of the hypothalamus. The *posterior choroidal arteries*, two or three on each side, arising as rami of the posterior cerebral artery, curve round the midbrain to enter the third ventricle's choroid plexus via the transverse fissure, supplying the adjacent tectum and the superior part of the thalamus.

Posterior cranial fossa

The brainstem and cerebellum are supplied by the vertebral and basilar arteries.

Distribution of the vertebral artery

Small *meningeal branches* supply the dura mater.

Two *posterior spinal arteries*, from the vertebral artery or its posterior inferior cerebellar branch, descend on each side behind the dorsal nerve roots, reinforced by intervertebral radicular arteries (*see* p. 227). They also supply the dorsal region of the closed part of the medulla, including the gracile and cuneate nuclei.

A single *anterior spinal artery* is formed by two tributaries, one from each vertebral artery, uniting in front of the medulla; as it descends in the cord's ventral median fissure it is augmented by the radicular arteries. Near its commencement it supplies the paramedian medullary region, including the pyramids, medial lemnisci and hypoglossal nerves (*see* p. 90).

Each *posterior inferior cerebellar artery*, the largest branch of the vertebral artery, winds round the olive's caudal end, ascending behind the vagal and glossopharyngeal roots, and descending along the fourth ventricle's lateral border and laterally into the vallecula cerebelli. This tortuosity may partly explain its susceptibility to thrombosis, but this may be secondary to occulsion of the parent vertebral artery. The vertebral arteries are usually unequal in size; sometimes one is much narrower. The cerebellar distribution is to the inferior vermis, inferolateral surface of the hemisphere and to the fourth ventricle's choroid plexus. En route the artery supplies the lateral medullary region, dorsal to the olive and lateral to the hypoglossal nerve. This includes the spinothalamic tracts, spinal trigeminal nucleus, nucleus ambiguus, visceral efferent pathway, nucleus solitarius, dorsal vagal, vestibular and cochlear nuclei, and the inferior cerebellar peduncle. Occlusion causes a 'lateral medullary syndrome' (*see* p. 92).

Distribution of the basilar artery

The basilar branches are bilateral and symmetrical (*Fig.* 14.2), and include numerous small *pontine arteries*.

Paired *anterior inferior cerebellar arteries* supply the anterior and inferior cerebellar cortex and white matter and also give off small medullary and pontine branches.

Each *labyrinthine artery*, arising directly from the basilar artery or from its anterior inferior cerebellar branch, accompanies the facial and vestibulocochlear nerves into the internal acoustic meatus, supplying the membranous labyrinth.

Each *superior cerebellar artery*, arising near the end of the basilar artery, is separated from the posterior cerebral artery by the oculomotor nerve, curving round the cerebral peduncle with the trochlear nerve. It ramifies over the superior cerebellar surface, supplying the cortex and white matter, including the central nuclei. It gives branches to the superior cerebellar peduncle, superior colliculus and pons.

Paired *posterior cerebral arteries*, forming the terminal basilar bifurcation, are distributed as described above (p. 223).

VENOUS DRAINAGE OF THE BRAIN

All venous drainage is to the dural venous sinuses (*see* Chapter 13). Veins from the brainstem and cerebellum enter adjacent sinuses in the posterior cranial fossa. The cerebrum has external and internal venous networks. The external veins are sub-arachnoid; the internal veins, draining deep structures and the choroid plexuses, emerge from the transverse fissure.

External cerebral veins

The *superior cerebral veins* ascend over the dorsolateral surfaces of the cerebrum, pierce the arachnoid mater, traverse the subdural space and enter the superior sagittal sinus or its lacunae. Traumatic anteroposterior displacement of the cerebral hemispheres may rupture these veins in the subdural cleavage plane, causing a subdural haemorrhage.

A *superficial middle cerebral vein* in each lateral fissure drains forwards to the cavernous sinus, is connected to the superior sagittal sinus by a *superior anastomotic vein* and to the transverse sinus by an *inferior anastomotic vein*.

A *deep middle cerebral vein* drains each insula, runs forward deep in the lateral fissure and is joined by an *anterior cerebral vein* to form a *basal vein*, which arches round the cerebral peduncle to enter the great cerebral vein.

Internal cerebral veins

A *thalamostriate vein* arises in the roof of each inferior ventricular horn, runs along the medial side of the tail and body of the caudate nucleus to unite with the *choroidal vein* near the interventricular foramen, to form an *internal cerebral vein* (*Fig.* 14.6). The two internal cerebral veins run posteriorly near the midline in the tela choroidea to the transverse fissure, uniting beneath the splenium as the *great cerebral vein* (of Galen), which is joined by the basal veins before entering the commencement of the straight sinus.

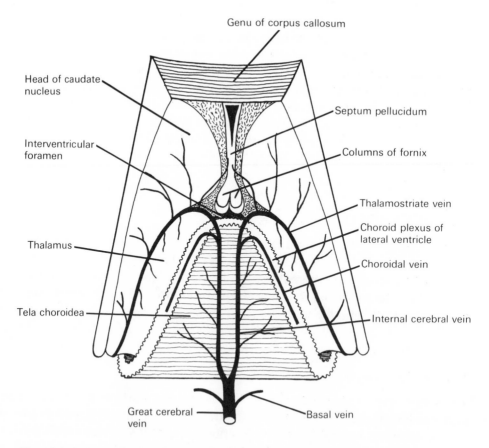

Fig. 14.6 A dissection of the internal cerebral veins and tela choroidea viewed from the posterosuperior aspect. The body and crura of the fornix have been removed.

BLOOD VESSELS OF THE SPINAL CORD

An *anterior spinal artery* and paired *posterior spinal arteries* descend throughout the cord in the pia mater, reinforced by multiple *radicular arteries* (from the vertebral, deep cervical, posterior intercostal, lumbar and sacral vessels). The latter traverse the intervertebral foramina, run medially to the cord along the ventral and dorsal spinal roots to join the longitudinal spinal vessels. They are the major supply to the spinal cord below the cervical region. In the lower thoracic or upper lumbar region, usually on the left, one radicular artery, the *arteria radicularis magna*, is particularly large and its occlusion may cause neural dysfunction. The posterior spinal arteries supply the dorsal grey and white columns; the rest of the cord is supplied by the anterior spinal artery.

The *veins of the spinal cord* follow the arterial pattern, draining by radicular veins to an extradural *internal vertebral venous plexus* which drains through the intervertebral foramina to the vertebral, posterior intercostal, lumbar and sacral veins. This extradural plexus has no valves, and infection or malignant tumours may spread in it. Since it communicates with the dural venous sinuses through the foramen magnum, prostatic or mammary tumours or a pleural abscess may thus spread to the brain.

APPLIED ANATOMY

CEREBRAL ARTERIAL OCCLUSION. This commonly results from the embolism of a blood clot, usually associated with arterial degeneration (atherosclerosis) in which a thrombus developing on damaged intima becomes detached. Atherosclerotic occlusion may occur in the carotid or vertebral vessels in the neck or cranium. Embolism occurs less often in heart disease: in mitral stenosis a clot may form in the left atrium; in coronary ischaemia there may be a 'mural thrombus'; in bacterial endocarditis 'vegetations' on mitral or aortic valves may be detached. Rarely, in severe fractures, fat globules are swept into the circulation and may lodge in the cerebral vessels.

The extent and pattern of nervous dysfunction depends on whether obstruction is in a main vascular trunk or confined to the central or cortical branches.

As the main continuation of the internal carotid artery, the *middle cerebral artery* is most commonly invaded by emboli. Obstruction of its trunk produces such widespread cerebral ischaemia and oedema that death may result. Thrombosis in the *cortical branches* of the dominant hemisphere causes contralateral paralysis of the upper limb and lower facial muscles, with inability to speak or write and, if the language area (of Wernicke) is involved, difficulty in understanding words. Damage on the non-dominant side causes facial and upper limb paralysis but no sensory or motor aphasia. Obstruction of the *central supply* (lateral striate vessels) to the internal capsule produces contralateral paralysis of the upper and lower limbs (hemiplegia); partial recovery involves flexor muscles of the arm and extensor muscles of the leg. The nuclei of many cranial nerves have some degree of bilateral cortical connexion and are either only partly affected or unaffected. In 'pseudobulbar palsy', phonation, mastication and deglutition are seriously impaired because of previous asymptomatic vascular deprivation of cortico-bulbar fibres in the contralateral internal capsule. Note that the lower facial muscles have a contralateral cortical innervation, the upper facial muscles a bilateral one.

Occlusion of *cortical* branches of the *posterior cerebral artery* results in contralateral visual field defects. The *central* arteries, including the posteromedial group and the posterior choroidal vessels, are clinically termed 'thalamogeniculate': damage to them causes hemianaesthesia and hemianopia; sensation is affected at thalamic level and recovery may be marred by severe intractable pain. Rarely, an obstructed central supply to the subthalamus produces hemiballismus, violent flailing movements in the contra-lateral limbs.

Thrombosis of the *anterior cerebral artery* is uncommon. Deprivation of the *cortical* supply results in paralysis and impaired sensation in the contralateral lower limb (paracentral lobule) and reduced awareness of it (superior parietal lobule). Occlusion of the *central* branches to the internal capsule is rare and produces contralateral weakness of the face and arm.

Since the *anterior choroidal artery* supplies the posterior limb of the internal capsule, retrolentiform area (optic radiation) and hippocampal formation, its obstruction may cause hemiparesis, hemianaesthesia, hemianopia and defective memory of recent events.

INTRACRANIAL HAEMORRHAGE. *Extradural haemorrhage* usually follows direct blows in the temporal region, with fracture of the squamous temporal bone. Typically there is transient unconsciousness due to concussion, then a lucid interval, followed by signs of progressively raised intracranial pressure, leading to coma as blood accumulates between the skull and dura mater. Untreated, this may be fatal within a few hours.

Subdural haemorrhage follows sudden anteroposterior movement of the brain relative to the cranium. Rupture of a superior cerebral vein produces a subdural extravasation, but this may be small as the vein seals itself. A 'chronic subdural haematoma' then becomes surrounded by a fibrinous semipermeable membrane. Thus encapsulated, it slowly enlarges, producing headache, confusion and disturbance of memory–symptoms which may develop months after the original, often minor, incident.

Subarachnoid haemorrhage, usually due to rupture of a congenital aneurysm near the circulus arteriosus, causes sudden severe headache, nausea and vomiting, possibly followed by coma and death.

Cerebral haemorrhage, usually associated with hypertension, most frequently involves a lateral striate branch of a middle cerebral artery. If it is limited, there may be partial recovery with residual hemiplegia, due to damage of the internal capsule; extensive bleeding through the cortex or into the ventricles is fatal.

Chapter 15

Neurotransmitter pathways of the central nervous system

During the past twenty years advanced histochemical and neuroanatomical methods of investigation have been developed and applied to the nervous system. Initially the objective was to localize neurotransmitters at a cellular level through histochemical identification of either the neurotransmitter itself or one of its characteristic synthesizing enzymes. Techniques include fluorescence histochemical methods for monoamines, autoradiography for γ-aminobutyric acid (GABA) and immunohistochemistry using antisera raised against peptides or transmitter-synthesizing enzymes. More recently, histochemical methods have been combined with sophisticated tract-tracing techniques in order to define the projections of a neuron of known transmitter identity. Axon terminals take up an injected protein such as horseradish peroxidase (HRP) or a fluorescent dye such as Evan's Blue and transfer it by retrograde axonal transport to the soma, where it accumulates. Horseradish peroxidase can there be demonstrated by a simple enzyme histochemical technique, the fluorescent dyes by appropriate ultraviolet irradiation. Both the histochemical and tract-tracing methods have been adapted for electron microscopy, resulting in greater resolution and accuracy of observation.

Investigation has demonstrated neuron systems which utilize specific neuro-transmitters. Pioneering work carried out on small rodents is now being confirmed by examination of human post-mortem nervous tissue. This rapidly developing branch of neuroanatomy has considerable pharmacological significance and is briefly surveyed here.

MONOAMINE SYSTEMS

Included here are the catecholamines noradrenaline, dopamine and adrenaline and the indoleamine serotonin (5–HT). These were first located in reticular neurons by fluorescence techniques and more recently by using specific antisera and immunohisto-chemical detection. Transmitter-synthesizing *enzymes* peculiar to certain monoamine neuron systems can also be identified in this way. Thus tyrosine hydroxylase indicates the presence of noradrenaline or dopamine neurons. Identification of adrenaline neurons has resulted from immunohistochemical studies employing antisera raised against phenylethanolamine-*N*-methyl transferase (PNMT), the specific enzyme that methylates noradrenaline in adrenaline formation and is exclusive to adrenaline-containing neurons.

Noradrenaline neurons and pathways

There are several groups of noradrenaline neurons in the brainstem; their axons are long and they branch into extensive terminal networks. They form two main systems, the locus caeruleus and the lateral tegmental.

The *locus caeruleus* is a pigmented nucleus, ventromedial to the trigeminal mesencephalic nucleus, located mostly in the pons and extending into the midbrain. It consists entirely of noradrenaline neurons and these comprise almost half the total number in the central nervous system. The extensive projections of this nucleus are mostly ipsilateral in distribution. The major ascending pathway is termed the *dorsal catecholamine bundle*. It enters the midbrain tegmentum ventrolateral to the periaqueductal grey matter, turns ventrally to join the medial forebrain bundle and passes thence through the lateral hypothalamus to the septal area. As it ascends, the dorsal catecholamine bundle gives branches to the superior and inferior colliculi, dorsal raphé nuclei, habenular nuclei and the anterior, intralaminar and lateral geniculate thalamic nuclei. Terminal branches innervate the septal area and join the cingulum to be distributed to the entire neocortex. Other branches pass to the amygdala, hippocampus and subiculum. Within the cortex few fibres terminate in recognizable synapses; probably noradrenaline diffuses to small regions of cortical neurons. Other ascending projections from the locus caeruleus run in the dorsal longitudinal fasciculus to hypothalamic nuclei and in the central tegmental tract.

The locus caeruleus projects to the cerebellar cortex and intracerebellar nuclei via the superior cerebellar peduncle. Noradrenaline released from cortical terminals has a powerful inhibitory effect on Purkinje neurons. A descending pathway from the locus caeruleus innervates certain brainstem nuclei such as the dorsal vagal motor nucleus and trigeminal sensory nuclei. Thence it continues throughout the spinal cord, terminating in dorsal, lateral and ventral grey columns.

Through its extensive projections the locus caeruleus has a role in paradoxical sleep (*see* p. 203), cortical activation, facilitation and inhibition of sensory neurons and of preganglionic sympathetic neurons in the intermediolateral cell column of the spinal cord.

The *lateral tegmental system* comprises at least four groups of noradrenaline neurons, extending from the caudal medulla to a level rostral to the locus caeruleus in the midbrain. Their axons ascend in the central tegmental tract, traverse the diencephalon in the medial forebrain bundle and reach the septal area. This system contributes a major innervation to all the hypothalamic nuclei and to restricted regions of the thalamus. In contrast to the locus caeruleus system, distribution to the telencephalon is relatively limited and includes the olfactory region and amygdaloid nuclei. From the caudal medulla fibres descend to spinal grey matter.

The main functional significance of the lateral tegmental system is its noradrenaline innervation of the hypothalamus, particularly the medial nuclei and median eminence. Noradrenaline is apparently involved here in the regulation of the secretion of gonadotrophin, ACTH and growth hormone.

Dopamine neurons and pathways

Dopamine pathways are shorter than noradrenaline projections and have less extensive but very dense terminal fields of innervation. There are four main systems:

1. *Nigrostriate*. Dopamine neurons in the substantia nigra send axons to the caudate nucleus and putamen of the neostriatum. In Parkinson's disease (*see* p. 170) degeneration of this system severely reduces the dopamine concentration in the neostriatum and substantia nigra.
2. *Mesocortical (mesolimbic)*. The cells of origin of this system are located in the ventral tegmentum of the midbrain. Their axons ascend, enter the medial forebrain bundle and project to the limbic system. Excessive dopaminergic activity in this pathway simulates certain psychotic aspects of schizophrenia.
3. *Tubero-infundibular*. Axons from dopamine neurons in the arcuate nucleus and periventricular zone of the hypothalamus form this short tract which extends to the median eminence, infundibulum and hypophysis. Dopamine probably inhibits release of pituitary prolactin and luteinizing hormone releasing hormone (LHRH).
4. *Incertohypothalamic*. Axons from dopamine neurons in the zona incerta project to areas of the hypothalamus and may influence endocrine secretion.

Adrenaline neurons and pathways

The concentration of adrenaline in the central nervous system is much lower than that of other catecholamines. In the rostral medulla two groups of adrenaline neurons are present bilaterally in dorsomedial and ventrolateral positions and possibly also in relation to the nucleus solitarius and vagal dorsal motor nucleus. Axons of these adrenaline neurons terminate in the hypothalamus, in a number of visceral nuclei in the brainstem, in the locus caeruleus and in the intermediolateral cell column of the spinal cord. It is likely that they are involved in the integration of a wide range of visceral functions.

Serotonin (5–HT) neurons and pathways

Serotonin neurons are chiefly located in the midline raphé nuclei of the midbrain, pons and medulla oblongata. They have extensive projections throughout the brain and spinal cord, an arrangement comparable to noradrenaline pathways.

Ascending pathways

Most of these originate from mesencephalic and rostral pontine neurons. They give branches to the substantia nigra and interpeduncular nucleus, join the medial forebrain bundle and supply the posterior and lateral hypothalamic nuclei and the neostriatum. The most extensive distribution of these ascending fibres is to the limbic system; there is also a diffuse innervation of the neocortex via the cingulum. Ascending fibres modulate

behaviour. Destruction of serotonin neurons produces hypersensitivity to environ-
mental stimuli, hyperactivity and insomnia. Serotonin is involved in 'slow wave sleep'.
Lysergic acid diethylamide (LSD) depresses serotonin production and may produce
hallucinations; hence endogenous inhibition of serotonin production might, in theory,
result in mental disorder. The drug methysergide, a serotonin antagonist, is a potent
migraine prophylactic but its use is limited by potential side effects, particularly
retroperitoneal fibrosis.

Descending pathways

From raphé nuclei of the pons and medulla fibres descend in the dorsolateral spinal tract
to synapse with enkephalin-containing neurons of the substantia gelatinosa. Enkephalin
binds to opiate receptors of nociceptor afferent terminals, blocking impulse
transmission to the lateral spinothalamic tract (*Fig.* 4.11).

CHOLINERGIC SYSTEMS

Acetylcholine is widely distributed throughout the central nervous system. Early
attempts to localize cholinergic neurons employed, as a marker, the enzyme acetylcholinesterase (AChE), for which reliable enzyme histochemical methods were available.
However, following the discovery that AChE is not confined to cholinergic neurons, it
became urgent to develop a sensitive and reliable technique for the detection of choline
acetyltransferase (CAT) which is located only in cholinergic neurons. Only very
recently has an acceptable antiserum been raised against CAT for use in immuno-
histological studies. Thus the mapping of cholinergic systems in the central nervous
system, still in progress, is probably incomplete.

   CAT-positive neuron somata have been identified, as expected, in preganglionic
sympathetic neurons of the intermediolateral spinal column, in motor nuclei of the
ventral grey column and in cranial nerve nuclei with either a general somatic or a general
visceral efferent component.

Cholinergic pathways

1. *Habenulo-interpeduncular tract* (fasciculus retroflexus). This runs from the habenular
   nucleus of the epithalamus to the interpeduncular nucleus of the midbrain and is
   involved in autonomic control.
2. *Septohippocampal pathway.* From the septal area cholinergic fibres project via the
   fornix and fimbria to the hippocampus and adjacent subiculum, a reciprocal pathway
   in the limbic system.
3. *Cholinergic projections from the basal forebrain.* In the human forebrain there is
   an anteroinferior aggregation of magnocellular nuclei named the median septal
   nucleus, nucleus of the diagonal band, nucleus basalis and substantia innominata.
   These vary in their arrangement and may be collectively termed a 'magnocellular

basal nucleus'. Combined CAT immunohistochemistry and retrograde tracing techniques have shown that these nuclei provide a cholinergic innervation to the olfactory bulb, amygdala, hippocampus (*see* above) and also to the entire cerebral cortex. There are topographical relationships between individual nuclei and cortical regions. In Alzheimer's disease, a form of senile dementia, there is gross reduction of acetylcholinesterase and choline acetyltransferase in all these areas, few neurons in the nucleus basalis and depressed cholinergic innervation.

4. *Corpus striatum*. There are very high levels of acetylcholine in the neostriatum. Many intrinsic Golgi Type II neurons here are CAT-positive. In addition, some nigrostriate fibres are cholinergic and in Huntington's chorea (*see* p. 171) there is a decrease of choline acetyltransferase in the neostriatum.

GABA SYSTEMS

The concentration of γ-aminobutyric acid (GABA) in the central nervous system is much higher than that of acetylcholine or any of the monoamines. Its distribution is widespread; it is present in large numbers of neurons and may also be stored in glia. Its function is always that of inhibition. Of the many GABA neurons the most prominent are cerebellar (Purkinje, stellate, basket and Golgi cells), hippocampal, cortical and neostriatal interneurons. In Huntington's chorea there is degeneration of GABA neurons of the striatonigral pathway.

PEPTIDE SYSTEMS

For some decades peptides within the brain have been known to be associated with certain hypothalamic hormones and releasing factors. Since 1970 over twenty additional peptides, many of which were initially detected in the gut wall, have been found in neurons of the central and peripheral nervous systems. Peptides are widely distributed and detailed maps are available of enkephalin, substance P, somatostatin, neurotensin and cholecystokinin. There is strong evidence that *some* peptides such as substance P act as neurotransmitters, but the function of others is less clear. Moreover, peptides may co-exist in the same neurons as classical neurotransmitters such as dopamine, serotonin, noradrenaline and acetylcholine; their co-release on stimulation raises the possibility that some peptides may *modulate* the action of the classical neurotransmitters rather than being transmitters themselves.

The hypothalamus, amygdala, some brainstem nuclei and the dorsal grey column of the spinal cord are particularly rich in peptides; other areas such as the cerebellar cortex contain few. Peptides may occur both in Golgi Type I neurons, for example substance P in the habenulo-interpeduncular tract, and in Golgi Type II neurons, for example vasoactive intestinal polypeptide (VIP) in cortical interneurons. Substance P may be the neurotransmitter of certain primary sensory neurons mediating nociceptive sensations. Opioid peptides such as enkephalin modulate this input in endogenous analgesia (*see* p. 59). Peptide distribution and function form a rapidly expanding branch of neurobiological research.

Selected Bibliography

Brodal A. (1981) *Neurological Anatomy in Relation to Clinical Medicine*. Oxford, Oxford University Press.

Brodmann K. (1909) *Vergleichende Lokalisationslehre der Grosshirnrinde in ihren Prinzipien dargestellt auf Grund des Zellenbaues*. Leipzig, J. A. Barth.

Carpenter M. B. and Sutin J. (1983) *Human Neuroanatomy*. Baltimore, Williams & Wilkins.

Cotman C. W. (1978) *Neuronal Plasticity*. New York, Raven Press.

Cowan W. M. & Cuénod M. (1975) *The Use of Axonal Transport for Studies of Neuronal Connectivity*. Amsterdam, Elsevier.

Crosby E. C., Humphrey T. and Lauer E. W. (1962) *Correlative Anatomy of the Nervous System*. London, Macmillan.

De Robertis E. (1967) Ultrastructure and cytochemistry of the synaptic region. *Science*, **156**, 907–914.

Hubel D. H., and Wiesel T. N. (1974) Sequence regularity and geometry of orientation columns in the monkey striate cortex. *J. Comp. Neurol.*, **158**, 267–294.

Hubel D. H., Wiesel T. N. and LeVay S. (1977) Plasticity of ocular dominance columns in monkey striate cortex. *Phil. Trans. R. Soc. Lond. (Biol)*, **278**, 377–409.

International Nomenclature Committee (1977) *Nomina Anatomica*, 4th ed. Amsterdam, Excerpta Medica.

Kandel E. R. and Schwartz J. H. (1983) *Principles of Neural Science*. New York, Elsevier; London, Arnold.

Langley J. N. (1921) *The Autonomic Nervous System*. Cambridge, Heffer.

Melzack R. and Wall P. D. (1965) Pain mechanisms: a new theory. *Science*, **150**, 971–979.

Ottoson D. (1983) *Physiology of the Nervous System*. London, Macmillan.

Patten J. (1977) *Neurological Differential Diagnosis*. London, Starke; Heidelberg, Springer-Verlag.

Penfield W. and Rasmussen T. (1950) *The Cerebral Cortex of Man*. London, Macmillan.

Pert C. B., Snowman A. M. and Snyder S. H. (1974) Localization of opiate receptor binding in synaptic vesicles of rat brain. *Brain Res.*, **70**, 184–188.

Reynolds D. V. (1969) Surgery in the rat during electrical analgesia induced by focal brain stimulation. *Science*, **164**, 444.

Sarnat H. B. and Netsky M. G. (1975) *Evolution of the Nervous System*. Oxford, Oxford University Press.

Sinclair D. C. (1967) *Cutaneous Sensation*. Oxford, Oxford University Press.

Warwick R. (1953) Representation of the extraocular muscles in the oculomotor nuclei of the monkey. *J. Comp. Neurol.*, **98**, 449–504.

Warwick R. and Williams P. L. (1975) *Functional Neuroanatomy of Man*. London, Saunders.

Index